THE
HAPPY
COMMUTER

OVER 100 WAYS TO IMPROVE
AND ENJOY YOUR COMMUTE

MELISSA ADDEY

Dedicated to Ryan, who always knows the best route to take; and also to the Victoria Line on the London Underground, where I studied for my Masters.

Wherever you go, go with all your heart.

Confucius

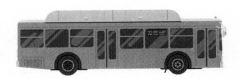

Table of Contents

Commuting is bad for you: why I wrote this book

<hr>

COMMUTING IS BAD FOR YOU. *Really* bad for you. If you commute for over 45 minutes each way every day, you are more likely to be overweight, suffer from anxiety, stress, depression and social isolation. You are more likely to sleep badly and be exhausted, have high blood sugar (which could lead to diabetes), high blood pressure and cholesterol (which could lead to heart attacks) and experience neck and back pain. You may have lower life satisfaction and happiness than people who do not commute. You may suffer from road rage if you drive or you may sit on a train every day reading negative news stories, which have been proven to make you sadder and more anxious, as well as more likely to exacerbate your own personal worries and anxieties. Oh, and you are 40% more likely to get divorced.*

There are over 500 million commuters in the world. If you commute 45 minutes per day in each direction, that's an hour and a half. Times five days a week, times 40 weeks a year (aren't I kind, giving you that many weeks' holiday?), times maybe 40 years of your working life? That's 12,000 hours of your life or 3 whole waking years.

When I read these statistics my first thought was: something needs to change. My second thought was: how can your commute be made better? This book is my attempt to answer that question. It focuses on taking back control of your

<hr>

commute and finding ways to make it a positive part of your life instead of something to be borne in misery.

*If you'd like to read up on the details of these studies, I've listed their sources at the end of the book.

People think my life has been tough, but I think it has been a wonderful journey. The older you get, the more you realise it's not what happens, but how you deal with it.

Tina Turner

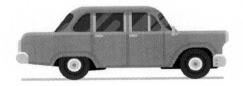

Is this book for you?

For this book to work best for you, I'm assuming that you are mostly commuting daily by train, metro, bus or car (as either a passenger or a driver). You may also be a very frequent traveler for work, in which case, welcome aboard. This book was written for all of you. Obviously some of the ideas don't work for people commuting by car - please don't read a book while driving! - but wherever possible I've tried to find a version of the idea that would work for drivers too, like audio books. I have also had readers suggest that of course this book might work for you any time you have to sit still a lot: waiting rooms, extended hospital stays, general travel and so on.

If you walk, cycle, drive a motorbike or paddle a canoe to work then this book is probably not for you. Studies show that more active commuters (e.g. people who cycle to work) are generally much happier than those who use more sedentary forms of transport – so you're probably a pretty happy commuter already. You may also need to pay more attention to your surroundings to keep safe and you may not have both hands available.

I'm guessing if you're reading this that your commute is not the best part of your day. I hope this book can help you improve your journey. There are lots of ideas you can try out, as well as making permanent shifts in your overall approach and attitude to commuting.

Come on, let's get going.

You know more of a road by having traveled it than by all the conjectures and descriptions in the world.

William Hazlitt

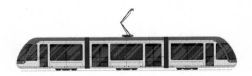

Changing your commuting attitude

A s a way of showing you how changes to your commute – and most importantly, your attitude towards commuting – can transform your experience, I'm going to use my own commuting experiences over the years.

I used to hate my commute. It was over an hour each way on a hot crowded London Underground train. There was never a seat to be had and I had a pretty handbag that slipped off my shoulder if I tried to hold a book. It never occurred to me to get a small backpack or that if I had traveled just three stops *away* from my destination to a quieter station and then come back up, I'd have had a seat with less than ten minutes' delay to my journey and at no extra cost.

I moved house. I was now based right at the last stop on my line, so there was always a seat to be had, at least in the mornings. And at the same time I started studying for my Masters degree and I did most of that studying on the commute into work, when I was still fresh and had a guaranteed seat. Now I saw my commute as a place to think, to develop new ideas, to plan my next essay. I gained a valuable qualification as a result of my commute to work – and freed up my weekends and evenings from a lot of studying that would otherwise have been done at those times.

I changed job, to one that allowed me to manage my own

time: amazing! When I did travel, I chose my times to do so and I avoided the rush hour if at all possible, which made a big difference. The train became a lovely place – plenty of seats, relaxed people around me, arriving at my destination calm and ready for work. I read lots of books, I listened to music, I wrote to-do lists.

I had a baby. Even in rush hour, the commute suddenly became my own personal 'me time'. I could get a cup of coffee and a croissant, settle down with a novel and enjoy nobody tugging at me wanting either attention or a bite of my croissant. Bliss.

Now I work from home. It's heaven. I am hardly ever on the train, and when I am it is for pleasure or an enjoyable part of business. I almost never hit the rush hour and when I do it almost feels like a novel experience because I know it won't last long and it won't be happening to me again for quite some time!

One of the common findings in studies about commuting is that **it is the loss of control in our lives that we find stressful.** We feel trapped in our commutes. We grow angry because we feel forced into them. We feel that our time has been hijacked by work and that our own time has somehow become our employer's time. But your commute is *yours*. It is your time and you *can* choose to change your experience of it. At some point in the past, you chose where to work and where to live. You chose which mode of transport to use. You chose what activities to do while you travelled. You chose what time to leave the house and what time you expected to be home. And you can alter all of those choices. Those commuters who felt that they were in control of their commute felt better than those who did not. Take the time to change your attitude to your commute and you may regain control and feel a whole lot better.

First of all, accept that you are in control.

Secondly, choose to reclaim your commute as *your* time.

Thirdly, decide how to make your commute the best it can possibly be: from tiny changes to really big shifts.

I travel light. I think the most important thing is to be in a good mood and enjoy life, wherever you are.

Diane von Furstenberg

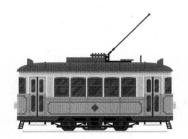

Get comfortable

BEFORE WE START LOOKING AT anything else about your commute, let's just get you comfortable on the commute you're already doing. Some of this section may seem obvious but I'm including it because for every idea I suggest, I have seen someone doing it wrong – or more likely, have done it wrong myself.

It is better to travel well than to arrive.

Buddha

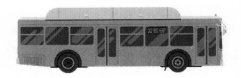

Get rid of the weight

PACK LIGHT. IT'S A CHALLENGE but not impossible and involves a good bag. I'm usually surprised at the stuff people are carrying with them on what would appear to be a normal day at work. Women in particular seem to carry a lot. I regularly see women carry: a pretty handbag which is unfortunately totally ruined by also carrying a large ugly sports bag which contains their gym kit plus quite often a plastic carrier bag stuffed to bursting with other mysterious necessities. There may come a moment in your life when you suddenly realise you can't go on like this: when you have kids and need to be hands-free, for example, or when your back starts giving you warning signals that it can't keep up. You need to pack differently. Pack like people off to climb Mount Everest: every tiny gram counts.

Use three steps to reduce your baggage. First of all: are you sure you need it at all? Secondly, check what you could leave at your workplace (or in your car): do you have a drawer in which you could leave the spare hosiery, tissues, extra tie, gym shoes, cute tiny handbag etc.? Thirdly: miniaturise. I've seen some very clever items out there: a hairbrush/mirror combo that is the size of a tiny compact, some very small umbrellas (they are not a bad size once opened, honest!), foldable water bottles and much more. Look at the contents of your bag that you really need and see if you can find a tiny version. I challenge you. Finally: choose a proper bag. A cutesy handbag or an oh-so-stylish manbag are no good if they are not big enough for the task in hand. Either invest in a really good classic bag (like a beautiful leather tote or briefcase) or acknowledge that practicality matters most and buy a proper, comfortable, backpack: it will take more stuff, leave your hands free, not ruin your back by dangling off one shoulder and at least look neat and organized, if not beautiful. More and more companies are making really nice backpacks now, so get one that is right for you and your journey. You should not carry more than one bag (unless you're going to very neatly spread the weight between two bags and have one on each side) and it should not be ruining your back!

If you drive, get rid of the junk in your car. Clear out the various odds and ends that have been slowly accumulating and give it a good clean. Then get something that keeps your stuff tidy when you're in the car. You'll feel better if your car is clean and tidy and you'll know where all your stuff is when you need it. And miniaturising works well for everyone, no matter how you get to work. (You could always choose a really tiny commuting car I suppose, it would make parking a lot easier!). Make sure you have a proper hands-free device for calls and get a decent music player or work out how your smart phone functions as one. Have all the things you need for your journey close to hand and make sure you carry a breakdown kit.

> I get ideas about what's essential when packing my suitcase.

Diane von Furstenberg

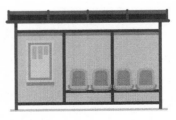

Adjust the temperature
(or dress right for it)

T OO HOT OR TOO COLD? Make sure you are wearing the right clothes (use layers if needs be) and take account of your surroundings. Some trains and planes pump viciously cold air at you while metro trains generally feel like the Sahara on a particularly hot day: so dress accordingly. Carry a fan with you (electric or handheld) for the hot days and have an extra layer for the cold days. Always carry even a small bottle of water. If you have a car, get the air conditioning fixed. Work out how to adjust the settings properly. Adjust it every day according to the weather.

It was one of those March days when
the sun shines hot and the wind blows
cold: when it is summer in the light,
and winter in the shade.

Charles Dickens

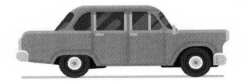

Slow down

ROAD RAGE OFTEN HAPPENS BECAUSE people are late for work and get more and more frustrated by inevitable traffic holdups. I see people rushing on the metro quite often – running down flights of stairs or escalators, dashing for the doors and getting caught in them and so on. London Underground says that this is how most people get hurt while traveling and runs an ongoing campaign urging people to take their time. Take their advice and leave a realistic amount of time for your commute: rushing is only likely to give you a few extra minutes anyway but can spoil your whole day by making you stressed. Prepare your clothes and breakfast the night before, get the kids' school stuff ready and lunchboxes packed. Yes, it's boring but you can do it with half an eye on a TV programme or while listening to music or chatting to your partner, housemates or kids, making it more enjoyable than doing the same tasks at breakneck speed in the mornings and then being annoyed because you are late, *again*. This might even give you time to apply your makeup at home rather than on the train, to eat your breakfast in your home instead of bolting it while standing up on a busy train or spilling your coffee in the car. Give yourself the gift of time and reduce some of the stress of commuting.

Everywhere, people are discovering that doing things more slowly often means doing them better and enjoying them more. It means living life instead of rushing through it. You can apply this to everything from food to parenting to work.

Carl Honore

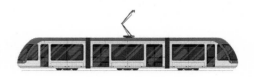

Cut down your costs and enjoy better food and drink

COMMUTING IS AN EXPENSIVE BUSINESS. You pay for tickets, for fuel, for your morning coffee and breakfast, for your lunch. Various studies show that people can easily spend £2,500 a year just on coffee and sandwiches and that commuting costs can use up as much as one-sixth of your wages. £2,500 sounds like a nice holiday or two to me! See what food and drink you can take from home to cut down on these costs and use the money you would have spent on something more fun. Supermarkets have an ever-increasing range of food that is easy to take along to work, from little porridge pots to fresh soups and salads. Or you can make your own. I used to have a box of porridge sachets in the office and make myself a nice hot breakfast when I got to work. My husband bought some quality ground coffee and a little cafetiere to keep in the office for his morning dose of caffeine. I've seen blenders that come with special glasses so that you can carry your freshly-made smoothie to work with you. There's every kind of pretty commuter cups, cool lunchboxes and soup-drinking thermos cups available, so invest in some good equipment, find some food and drink solutions you're happy with and you'll be saving money, eating better and more healthily. *Bon appétit!*

I would never be able to lead the insane lifestyle I do, traveling all over the world, if I wasn't eating food that was simple and healthy.

Alain Ducasse

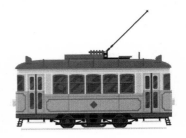

Stretch your mind

L ET'S FACE IT, ON A commute you've made about a million times before, you're using very little of your brain power. Zombies is the word that springs to mind when watching commuters getting on and off trains, turning left or right in that dazed way that means they're hardly thinking about what they're doing at all. A little more effort is required if you're driving a car, of course, but still: your commute could be a great opportunity to give your brain cells a workout. What knowledge do you feel is lacking in your life? Given my poor grasp of world geography I could probably do with staring at a map of the globe on any travels I undertake. As it was, I studied for my Masters on the London Underground and it made my commute a lot more interesting, as well as freeing up my home time when I would otherwise have had to study. Your commute is a wonderful opportunity to expand your knowledge. You can study for a qualification or undertake some personal development that you feel the need for: from revising for exams to reading up on baby books if you're expecting, how to fix a car to looking through books of great art.

We don't receive wisdom; we must discover it for ourselves after a journey that no one can take for us or spare us.

Marcel Proust

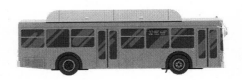

Do nothing at all

THERE'S SO MUCH TO DO in life and here I am suggesting still more things! You've looked after everyone else's needs, you have a full day of work ahead of you, when you get home there's more to do... so enjoy doing and thinking nothing at all. This way of using your commute probably really kicks in when you have kids or a lot on at work or at home and the idea of just sitting still, with no demands on you, with nothing at all to do for the next hour is bliss. Enjoy doing nothing. Relax, close your eyes if possible, let your mind drift and enjoy the stillness. We all need a bit of it sometimes.

The real test of friendship is: can you literally do nothing with the other person? Can you enjoy those moments of life that are utterly simple?

Eugene Kennedy

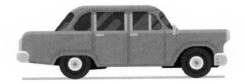

Learn a language

C HOOSE A LANGUAGE THAT YOU need to refresh or start from scratch with one you've always wanted to learn. Perhaps you need a new language for work. My sister studied Spanish intensively for 200 hours and by the end of it could comfortably read it and hold conversations. That's about half a year of commuting – not bad! You can use language courses on CD and as downloads, get yourself a pen pal (or email pal, more likely) to improve your reading and writing skills, watch foreign language films with subtitles to help you along in the beginning and listen to songs in your chosen language. If you are able to hold conversations by phone while you commute by car you might be able to improve your conversation skills with a teacher. Plan a holiday to a country that uses the language and find apps, games, TV shows and books that you can use on your commute to strengthen your new skill. Flashcards can also be a good tool while travelling. Look out the window and describe what you're seeing in your head in the new language.

I speak two languages: Body and English.

Mae West

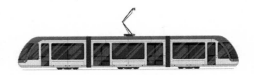

Enter competitions

I'M NOT GOING TO SUGGEST that you can pack in the day job by entering competitions, but a lot of people enjoy 'comping' as a hobby and end up winning a range of prizes from a new pair of gardening gloves to TVs and holidays. Look around for some good tips so that you don't end up following scams. Regular 'compers' set up a separate email address to use on entry forms so that they are not inundated by spam, and use a piece of (free) software to automatically enter their personal details into entry forms. If you get into the habit and spend your commute every day entering competitions, you're likely to pick up some nice prizes over time. Always a bonus!

Show class, have pride, and display character. If you do, winning takes care of itself.

Paul Bryant

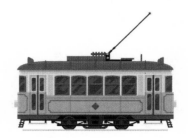

Take surveys for rewards

T HERE ARE QUITE A FEW online organisations that will pay you (again, it's just a bit, don't get over-excited!) to give your opinion on a range of subjects, through taking surveys. They set up surveys for which you usually earn points, which get turned into cash or high street voucher payouts when you've earned enough. There are also growing opportunities to be an online 'mystery shopper' – checking that websites are easy to navigate and so on. Again, do your homework before signing up with some reputable organisations and earning a little extra something to go shopping with.

I think somebody ought to do a survey as to how many great, important men have quit to spend time with their families who then spent any more time with their family.

Walter Cronkite

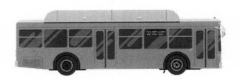

Deconstruct adverts

SOUNDS FANCY BUT REALLY, YOU probably do this all the time. Take a look at an advert on the train, billboard or platform where you find yourself. Is it being fully truthful? Does it have some strange suggestions or products? Who is backing it and what are they trying to sell you? I've seen some pretty odd ones, such as nutritionists telling me such-and-such a product is really good for me, only to notice they are employed by the gigantic company that makes said product. Hmmm. Or the advert I saw suggesting that you could easily have an extra-marital affair if you just kept your wife sweet by buying her the item being advertised: I actually complained about that one as did a lot of other people and it got withdrawn...

Advertising is the art of convincing people to spend money they don't have for something they don't need.

Will Rogers

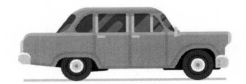

Be nosy

P EOPLE WATCHING IS A WONDERFUL pastime and on transport you can often elevate it into an art form. There are lots of people around you, usually wrapped up in their own thoughts and frequently forgetting what they look like to other people. Look at other people's gardens, through people's windows, into their cars (you see a lot going on in other people's cars) and more. While you may spot people nose-picking and other yucky habits, you may also get great fashion ideas, take a look at how they are passing their time (let me know if you spot any good ideas) and wonder about their lives as your commutes intersect for a brief moment. People's private phone calls can also be unintentionally quite amusing.

For me, one of the privileges of being a writer is to poke your nose around and learn about worlds you don't know.

Gavin Hood

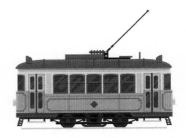

Tune into the radio

M ANY PEOPLE HAVE THEIR OWN favourite programmes such as long-running soap operas or *Woman's Hour*, but there may be many aspects of radio you haven't yet explored: new dramas and wonderfully re-told classics, bookclubs, the news, cookery shows, comedy and of course music of every kind. You may have got stuck in a rut, always listening to the same radio stations, so branch out a little. Or radio generally may be quite new to you because you're more used to other forms of media, in which case it's a whole new world to explore. If you get into the radio you can also look out for podcasts from various sources. If you can't get a radio signal during part of your commute then you can often access programmes after they have gone out live via their online archive.

I started writing my own songs from the time I was a little kid. I would write my own lyrics to other people's songs that I heard on the radio and take whatever song and make it about fairies and angels - whatever little girls sing about.

Bonnie McKee

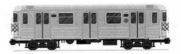

Change your worldview: TED

I LOVE TED, WHICH SHOWCASES INSPIRATIONAL thinkers and leaders from all over the world gathering to talk and share ideas. They have everything from musicians to jugglers, mathematicians to ecologists and orgasm experts. The talks last from under five minutes to well over half an hour so they can fit any length of commute. They will make you think about everything from enduring love to Stephen Hawking questioning the universe and everything in between, including why the way we think about work is 'broken' and how too many rules at work stop you getting things done... something to share with your boss when you get in, perhaps? Give them a go and see what gets you thinking differently or just enjoying something new. I've found things on TED that made me laugh out loud as well as fascinating new data that was useful for my workplace. Filling your commute with something mind-expanding can give you new ideas for work or refresh your mind after a long hard day.

Nothing is more dangerous than a dogmatic worldview - nothing more constraining, more blinding to innovation, more destructive of openness to novelty.

Stephen Jay Gould

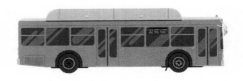

Get more creative

CREATIVITY IS BECOMING A SOUGHT-AFTER skill and you can develop yours by thinking of your brain as being made up of lots of little paths. If you think about going to work your brain will just go down its usual 'route' of whatever your normal way to work consists of. But if you think of a new way to go to work your brain will need to create a new pathway to take account of this new and surprising change. It's easy to let your thinking get routine, so a simple way to get more creative is to do routine things differently. Find a new route to work, pick up a newspaper you never usually read, arrive at your workplace via a different entrance and have a lunch you have never tried before.

You'll find over time that you will start to think of new ideas, make different connections and perhaps change your mind about a few things of which you were certain. Creativity is yours for the asking: just act differently and your brain will start to think differently as you give it new routes from which to choose solutions.

Creativity is putting your imagination to work, and it's produced the most extraordinary results in human culture.

Ken Robinson

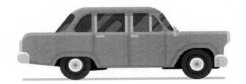

Do some colouring-in

THINK YOUR COLOURING-IN DAYS ARE long gone? I think not. A big new trend right now is for grown-up colouring books (and there are apps for this as well). Some are large format but I've also seen some handily pocket-sized versions. They have some truly beautiful and very complex designs for you to add your own creativity to, so get yourself one of these, a little pack of colouring pencils and return to your childhood. It's very enjoyable and relaxing to do. If you usually end up doodling in meetings, like I always do, then you'll probably love these.

I sometimes think that what I do as a writer is make a kind of colouring book, where all the lines are there, and then you put in the colour.

John Irving

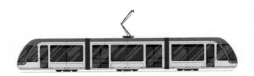

Visualise the future

WHAT DO YOU WANT FROM your life and how are you going to get it? Your commute is a great time to focus on this question. Spend some time dreaming up your ideal life. Yes, some of you might think of yachts, stunning partners and more cash than you know what to do with but everyone has their own unique ideal life fantasy. Some are more achievable than others but I think most people could at least edge their current life closer to their ideal. Allow yourself some real fantasy time and then note what are the main themes coming up over and over. Is it travel? A nice house? Wild adventure? You might like to use *The Desire Map*, by Danielle LaPorte, who helps you drill down from the material things into what those things are going to make you *feel* (comforted, relaxed, excited, etc.) rather than just *have* and see what you can do to make your visualisation come true, or at least truer.

We need not be afraid of the future,
for the future will be in our own hands.

Thomas Dewey

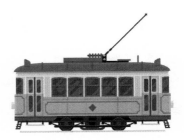

Let go of the past

P EOPLE MAY HAVE DONE MEAN things to you or things may have gone wrong – from minor to major. Let them go. Close your eyes (not if you're driving, folks!), review the past, whether yesterday or many years ago and then decide to move on. That was then and this is now and you can choose to let it go. Of course if you have suffered some serious traumas in the past you may need the help of a professional and therefore this activity will not be suitable for your commute, but many of us carry round small hurts, grievances and just plain annoyances for years without realising what a drain on our current life and energy they can be. Let go of that stuff: it's just not worth it. Feel better, stronger and happier without it.

Forget the past.

Nelson Mandela

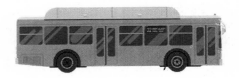

Use your imagination

"Hmm", I ponder. "Nope, not taking him along, he'd never climb a coconut tree. But her, yes, she looks promising. I bet she could spear a fish." This is my own silly game I play when traveling. I look round the train carriage and wonder which six people I would take with me to a desert island. Do they look like they're up to it? Do they look like they can climb trees or calm people down when things get tough and people start squabbling? Play your own games. Choose people or things you go past and invent games around them. Play murder mysteries, invent reality TV concepts, host dating gameshows and figure out your very own Hunger Games winners. It can be a lot of fun and makes you use your imagination in weird and wonderful ways. Build new buildings on empty plots you pass by and turn wastelands into the Hanging Gardens of Babylon. What if the apocalypse was tomorrow? Start planning. Food, shelter, protection? And so on. Plan your way out of the dinosaurs getting out of that theme park *again*, the zombies on the loose, the vampires coming after you (though they might be cute of course, who knows….). You get the drift. Since your imagination is going to be better than any game you can buy, I think you'll enjoy yourself once you get going. There is no restriction on your imagination and what it can do.

Think left and think right and think
low and think high. Oh, the thinks you
can think up if only you try!

Dr. Seuss

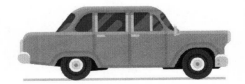

Sort out problems one small step at a time.

PROBLEMS AT WORK OR AT home can get overwhelming. Take the time when you are commuting and are 'outside' your normal life, to ponder small parts of the problems you are facing. Is there a small step you can take to make it a *little* better? And a bit better than that? Sometimes even small things make a difference to the overall problem or make it easier to bear. Find little ways to improve the situation and ease the burden.

Whoever wants to reach a distant
goal must take small steps.

Saul Bellow

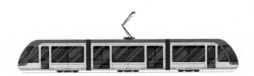

Learn some new words

NEVER MIND LEARNING NEW LANGUAGES, make the most of the one you've got. We're all guilty of sticking to a tiny vocabulary when there's an astonishing array of wonderful words to use out there. Learn one new word each day and then practice using it during your commute in your mind – and out loud once you get to work. You can get a dictionary, word-a-day calendars or apps for this exercise and if you're driving then of course you can look up the word before you leave the house and practice uses for it as you drive.

A new word is like a fresh seed sown
on the ground of the discussion.

Ludwig Wittgenstein

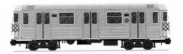

Give your brain
something to work on

THERE ARE SO MANY GAMES and apps designed to give your brain a workout, so try a few and see how you get on. The American Alzheimer's Association endorsed Sudoku as the kind of brain game that may stave off or improve the onset of the disease. Jigsaws or crossword puzzles can be fun and there are plenty of apps for them too. If you're feeling super-smart you can always try one of those 'test your IQ at home' exercises. I came out as a Mensa-level genius on one of those tests, although it's *possible* that I forgot to set the timer (ahem).

Keeping an active mind has been vital to my survival, as has been maintaining a sense of humor.

Stephen Hawking

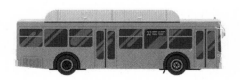

Keep up with current affairs

DON'T REMAIN IGNORANT OF WHAT'S going on in the world. Take a few moments each day to see what's happening around you, both locally (where perhaps you can act accordingly to improve a bad situation or benefit from something good) and on a wider scale around the world, to see great things that are happening and to realise that probably you are a very blessed person in relation to many others in our world. If you can think of a positive way to help, do so. I do think that the news errs heavily on the negative side though, so try not to weigh down your life with one negative story after another just because the news editor thinks that bad things happening makes a 'good story'.

It's amazing that the amount of news that happens in the world every day always just exactly fits the newspaper.

Jerry Seinfeld

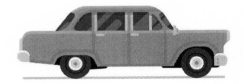

Prepare for the work ahead

O N YOUR WAY INTO WORK, take a little time to visualise the day ahead of you. Spot any tricky parts to the day and think about how to navigate them safely and positively. Think about the things you'd really like to achieve and prioritise things to do. This visualisation will help your day go more smoothly because you have already thought about how to deal with possible snags.

We cannot solve our problems with the same thinking we used when we created them.

Albert Einstein

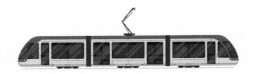

Close down your work day

O N YOUR WAY HOME THINK about how the day went. Give yourself a pat on the back for the stuff that went well and take a look at things that didn't quite go to plan. Is there something you can improve for tomorrow? Are there people to say thank you to for the good things? Have you learnt anything useful? Also, take a brief moment to 'close down' work, to focus on your home life and not drag your work life home with you. Some people never switch off and this is tiring for them and not great for family life. A few moments to let go of work for the day can be a great way to arrive home ready for a different part of your day.

Some of us think holding on makes us strong; but sometimes it is letting go.

Hermann Hesse

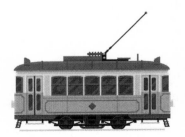

Keep a diary

A DIARY DOESN'T HAVE TO BE some work of literary genius, written on scented paper with a fountain pen. There are diaries that are just one line a day and many people keep diaries that have doodles, shopping lists, random phone numbers and other jottings along with their thoughts and a record of their lives. I have a friend who keeps a scrapbook-like diary of tickets for events she has attended over the years and so on. Find something to record your diary in – from a Dictaphone if you are driving to a pretty notepad and get started. Diaries can lead us to see more clearly the patterns of our lives and new directions emerging. My mother has written diaries all her life and has sometimes allowed me to read them, providing an unusual insight into another person's feelings and priorities that is illuminating, although of course most people prefer to keep their diaries private.

The moment I was introduced to my wife, Emma, at a party I thought, here she is - and 20 minutes later I told her she ought to marry me. She thought I was as mad as a rat. She wouldn't even give me her telephone number - and she wrote in her diary: "A funny little man asked me to marry him."

Julian Fellowes

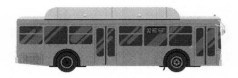

Memorise poems, songs and stories

P EOPLE DON'T REALLY DO THIS anymore, but memorising poems used to be something children did quite a lot and so as adults they would have many lovely poems in their memory banks, ready to be taken out and used to entertain themselves and others. My son's favourite so far is about a wicked cat called Macavity (T S Eliot), and of course your own choice will be very individual to you. If you've not had many dealings with poems until now, get an anthology of popular poems so that you can find a good starting point for your own favourites. Choose a poem you really like (however short) and memorise it. It can be fun to choose poems related to your surroundings. The London Underground has Poems on the Underground, where short poems are displayed in each train carriage, which is quite fun as you can spot your favourites and find some new gems. My mother could recite *The Lion and Albert* on long walks, which we children found hilarious. There are dramatic poems and funny poems, tender poems and sad poems, as well as poems about travelling which may be quite pertinent to you as you commute back and forth. You could also, of course, memorise stories, jokes and songs.

Poetry gives us courage and sets us straight with the world. Poems are great companions and friends.

David Whyte

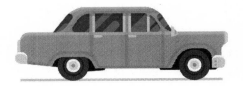

Draw what you can remember

A FRIEND OF A FRIEND HAS a novel approach to improving her memory. A keen artist, she thinks of a famous painting, then sketches everything she can remember of it, checking afterwards to see if she has included all the key elements. It uses her artistic skills, keeps her memory working and she finds it relaxing to think of paintings of which she is fond.

I dream of painting and then I paint
my dream.

Vincent Van Gogh

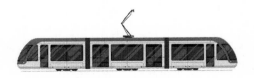

Look after your body

I N MOST OF THE STUDIES done, it seemed that commuters' bodies were taking the brunt of their commuting stress. So it might be worthwhile giving a little bit of extra tender loving care to your body while you travel. Yes, I know that unless you are a total exhibitionist sitting in a very empty train carriage you're unlikely to be able to do your regular gym workout but there's still a lot you can be doing to give your physical self a little extra love.

I try to be grateful for the abundance of the blessings that I have, for the journey that I'm on and to relish each day as a gift.

James McGreevey

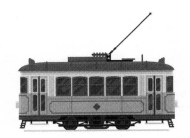

Eat

MOST PEOPLE WHO FAINT ON the London Underground do so during unexpected delays, especially when it's hot – and in particular after not having eaten breakfast. In the rush to get to work, many of us don't eat and our bodies, shaken awake and forced to hurry into the day's work, suffer as a result. If you can't eat breakfast at home, take something along with you. For example, a handful of nuts, an apple and a little bread roll would be a good start and very fast to grab as you rush out the door. Many of us don't eat enough fruit and vegetables. In the UK the recommended amount is five portions a day. Perhaps you could have two snacks each day, one on the way to work and one on the way home, each one being a portion – and in this way you'd already be two portions up on your current intake. Munch on an apple on the way in, eat a handful of carrot sticks on the way home and you'd be doing great. See which fruits and vegetables are portable and make this a new habit. You can even buy smoothie makers that have handy containers to carry your smoothie along with you. Some fruit, yoghurt and oats in a blender every morning could give you a wonderful start to the day in a matter of minutes. Leave the blender to soak if you don't have time to wash it straightaway so that it will be easy to clean later.

When a man's stomach is full it makes
no difference whether he is rich or
poor.

Euripides

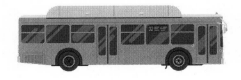

Drink

OUR PLANET COULD SERIOUSLY DO with less plastic water bottles floating about its seas, but your body could do with good hydration. Get yourself a really nice water bottle of your own with a sports cap for easy sipping and less accidental spillages. Fill it up every day from the tap or a water filter and drink a bottle on your way in and a bottle on your way back from work. I think you'll feel a real difference. You could also take along a juice (one more of your five a day) and cold herbal teas, or get a flask and have hot drinks on wintery days. As for something to kick start your day, get yourself a commuter's cup and make proper high quality tea or coffee at home to take along with you, or buy a good quality mini teapot or cafetiere and enjoy a hot drink when you get to work – you'll save money and have a much nicer drink on your journey.

Thousands have lived without love,
not one without water.

W. H. Auden

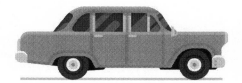

Sleep

THERE'S A GREAT CUSHION I saw recently made for long journeys, a kind of three-pronged shape, which not only supports your neck but also your jaw, so that you don't end up with your mouth open as you sleep, drooling over your fellow commuters and embarrassing yourself by snoring loudly. Grab one of these and set some kind of alarm for yourself (perhaps your phone on vibrate) so that you don't miss your stop, then catch up on some much needed sleep. If you commute for over an hour, this can make you feel a lot more refreshed if you have to get up early or if you do it on the way home you'll arrive back in good shape for a sociable evening with family or friends rather than exhausted and grumpy after a long day's work. If you're good at power naps then even 15 minutes or so will make a difference to how you feel for the rest of the day or evening.

It is a common experience that a problem difficult at night is resolved in the morning after the committee of sleep has worked on it.

John Steinbeck

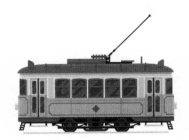

Exercise

YOU KNOW THE DRILL. TAKE the stairs and walk up the escalators. Whatever distance you walk, walk briskly and move your arms. Get out or park one stop early and walk the rest of the way. Walk up to your workplace instead of taking the elevator. If there are no seats to be had, practice improving your balance by only holding on lightly to a support, making your body work to stay upright – this is all that 'core' work is, after all. Wear weights on your wrists, ankles or even a weighted vest (you will look weird, but hey...). If you're sitting down then at least roll your neck and shoulders to loosen them up and for the women – work on the infamous pelvic floor. You can actually just tighten and loosen your muscles all over your body while sitting down – every little thing makes a difference. If you find yourself entirely alone in a London Underground train carriage with poles available, you could always work on your pole dancing moves and get some pull-ups done. Just saying...

Walking is the best possible exercise.
Habituate yourself to walk very far.

Thomas Jefferson

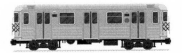

Exercise your face

I F RUNNING UP THE ESCALATORS sounds awful, then try out something simpler and less tiring: facial fitness. You can find face yoga, face fitness and face workouts to follow in DVDs, books and apps for your phone. Because you're toning up the muscles that support your facial skin, using these exercises is supposed to keep your face away from the need to Botox or similar: and really, it would be better to look like yourself (on a great day) rather than someone else... The exercises are fairly simple, for example 'the giraffe', which involves stretching your neck up really high (head tilted back a bit) and lightly stroking your neck skin downwards. Easy! Look up a few exercises and try out the ones you can do while commuting without looking *too* odd to your fellow commuters.

If you're paralysing your face in your 20s and 30s, you're not exercising the muscles that give it strength. My feeling is, laugh, cry, move your face.

Salma Hayek

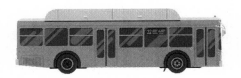

Pop your pills

I F YOU'RE SAT THERE WITH a bottle of water by your side (see the earlier point on being well hydrated) then you might want to add some pills to your next sip. Research what vitamins or supplements might be good for you and have them handy so you don't forget to take them. It's very easy to forget to take your vitamins especially if breakfast is eaten on the run or you forget to eat it at all (you need to go back and read the earlier point, I think!) but even a little extra care of yourself will make a big difference to your health and how you feel on a daily basis. No need to carry round lots of bottles - you can get a small pillbox in which to keep your daily doses. For example, 70% of adults in the UK are lacking in Vitamin D, which contributes to the proper absorption of calcium, amongst other minerals. Read up on what supplements might be useful for your own needs and keep them where you won't forget to take them. If you don't like taking supplements then think about what vitamins and minerals you might be in need of and see what you can eat to get them naturally, for example you could snack on a little handful of nuts to help grow stronger hair and nails.

Glamour is about feeling good in your own skin.

Zoe Saldana

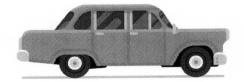

Cherish your body

T AKE A MOMENT TO THINK about the parts of your body you love the most, from your nicely shaped earlobes to your perfect feet. Then think about the parts of your body that you don't view with such enthusiasm and try to find good things about them. For starters, stretch marks may be the result of your body having created a baby, an extraordinary feat and one you can justly be proud of. Bit of a pot belly? Perhaps the result of a loving family who eat together and enjoy good food. Take every part of your body, from your hair down to your toenails and either see the beauty or find some, whatever it takes and however convoluted your reasoning. You'll be surprised at how positive an exercise this is. As an example, the women in my family are, ahem, *blessed* with marvellously sturdy ankles, but to be fair we are not known for twisting them either, which my husband, with his far more elegant specimens, does quite frequently. So maybe there is a positive reason for their solidity, despite their lack of superficial charm. My husband, of course, can count his ankles as things of beauty, even if they do twist occasionally! Find the good and the beauty in your own body and be grateful for it.

Body love is more than acceptance
of self or the acceptance of the
body. Body love is about self-worth in
general. It's more than our physical
appearance.

Mary Lambert

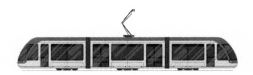

Relax

W<small>E ALREADY KNOW THAT COMMUTING</small> can be stressful. Time for some relaxation. This exercise simply relaxes one set of muscles at a time. Not completely of course or you'll be slumped in your seat like a jellyfish, but enough to let go of any stress you are holding onto. Start with your toes and feel them tense up, then let them relax. Move up to your foot and do the same. Do this exercise slowly and feel your whole body gradually relax and let go of tension. You will probably find along the way that you need to adjust your posture...

Melissa Addey

Your mind will answer most questions
if you learn to relax and wait for the
answer.

William S. Burroughs

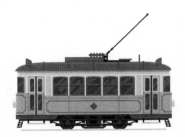

Sort out your posture

DRIVING, SITTING OR STANDING IN a crowded train – these are not likely to be developing a great posture for you. But bad posture, over time, can really cause pain, especially to your back. Try to take a moment each day during your commute, preferably at the start so you can benefit from it all the way, to really get your posture sorted out. Get your bottom or feet firmly planted, pull up to your full height so that your torso has room for your vital organs to function and your head feels as though a thread is pulling it upwards from the crown. Let your shoulders fall down. Try to keep a good posture throughout your journey. This will be hard at first but if you keep doing it you will feel a difference and your body will be grateful for it (and so will you when you don't get a fearsome backache).

I'd love to look like my mum when I am her age. She taught ballet for years, and my attitude to exercise and fitness has definitely been influenced by her. She's 84 now, and I've watched how well she has aged, and a lot of that is to do with her fantastic posture.

Sarah Parish

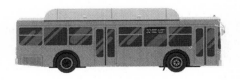

Get a seat

HAVING A SEAT ON A crowded train is a great joy and makes a considerable difference to your journey. You can relax more, you will be (marginally) less pressed up against other people and you can perhaps focus better on activities that distract your from your surroundings, like reading a good book. Try starting earlier, or doubling back so that you travel away from your destination a few stops to a quieter station where you can continue your journey in comfort.

If you work in a job with a lot of walking involved (around shops, factory floors and the like) then coming back home on a train with no seats available can be exhausting. If you don't care about getting some funny looks, consider taking a tiny, light, portable chair with you, of the kind fishermen use. When there's no seats left but it's not too crammed, pop out your little chair and settle down.

If you're in a car, then obviously you have a seat, but try to make sure it's a comfy one rather than putting up with that slightly awkward angle it seems to be set at or if you commute as a family to do school drop-offs and more, then try and find car seats for the kids that don't take up *all* the room, leaving people squashed. For drivers, you might want to upgrade your seat... perhaps a seat that gives you better orthopedic support might be nice. There are plenty to choose from and if you're going to be sat in a car for a long time it might make a real difference to how you feel when you get home.

If you are pregnant, make sure to wear a badge that

proclaims your condition as people may genuinely not notice you or be uncertain that you're pregnant especially in the early days (when you often feel awful but look your normal size). If you have a valid reason to need a seat, then please do ask someone. Often people just don't notice what's going on around them.

> Happiness is a butterfly, which when pursued, is always just beyond your grasp, but which, if you will sit down quietly, may alight upon you.
>
> Nathaniel Hawthorne

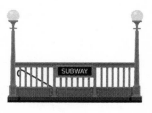

Spice up your sex life

G IVE YOUR BODY SOMETHING SEXY to look forward to by preparing yourself. Exercise your pelvic floor (no one will know you're doing it, honest) and read up on new moves to try out from the Kama Sutra or the (many!) other guides available. You can always buy the ebook or audio versions of these books if you'd rather everyone else didn't know what you're reading...

Take the time to send some sexy messages to your loved one and read or listen to erotica to get yourself in the mood.

Sex is a part of nature. I go along with nature.

Marilyn Monroe

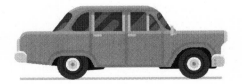

Relish a new perfume

I HAVE A FRIEND WHO IS a perfume fiend. Her bedroom has more bottles of scent than a department store and a new perfume is a source of interest and delight to her, especially when on a crowded (and less than fragrant) train. A little dab on the wrist in the morning is something to enjoy as you travel to work and make you feel fresh on the return journey.

Until I was a teenager, I used red pokeberries for lipstick and a burnt matchstick for eyeliner. I used honeysuckle for perfume.

Dolly Parton

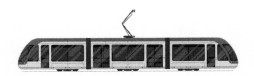

Enjoy a massage

P OSSIBLY STRIPPING DOWN TO YOUR underwear and having a massage might be frowned upon by your fellow commuters, even if you could find a masseuse willing to massage you on public transport or sit in the back seat of your car. But all is not lost. People are always getting massages for their backs, their heads, arms, legs, feet... but very rarely for their hands, one of the most extraordinary and hard-working parts of your body. So take a little bit of a simple cream, oil or even baby powder (it slips like oil but doesn't leave stains on your clothes) with you and massage your hands. Simple movements are fine, something akin to a really good washing of your hands but with more attention to how it feels and giving your fingers a good stretch and bend along the way. For drivers who shouldn't be taking their hands off the wheel, install a massaging seat-cover in your car and you'll get a back massage during your journey – perfect.

Melissa Addey

Massage therapy has been shown to relieve depression, especially in people who have chronic fatigue syndrome; other studies also suggest benefit for other populations.

Andrew Weil

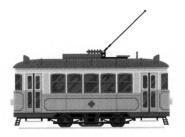

Moisturise

A GAIN, LET'S NOT GET TOO carried away. Now is not the time to rub in the stretch mark cream or the anti-cellulite miracle worker. But the skin on your hands is the most prone to looking old before its time (or just giving your real age away), so an extra application of moisturiser once a day could be very beneficial. If you need serious moisturising and don't mind looking a little odd, then put on lots of cream and pull gloves on over the top (you can probably best get away with this in winter!). An hour's soaking-in might do wonders. On your way home, if you're feeling a bit tired and frazzled, a facial spray might be in order: there are many of these so find one that suits you and your skin and give your face a nice energising boost.

The finest clothing made is a person's own skin, but, of course, society demands something more than this.

Mark Twain

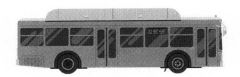

Breathe

THIS MAY SOUND STUPID BUT often we forget to breathe. Air is coming in and going out, but quite possibly in a substandard way, enough to keep us ticking over, not enough to make us feel great when we do it. Many commuting positions can easily lead to a slumped posture (as can so many other activities in life), so take a few moments to get into the habit of good breathing. If you start each commute with ten deep, long breaths you will feel better as slow, deep breathing also tends to relax people when they are stressed. So get your shoulders back and your head up, straighten your torso so the air has somewhere to go and get breathing. If you do this every time you commute it will take up a tiny amount of time and you will start to do it at other times too once you know how good it can make you feel.

When you arise in the morning, think of what a precious privilege it is to be alive - to breathe, to think, to enjoy, to love.

Marcus Aurelius

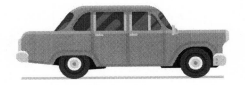

Plan a new wardrobe

THERE ARE TIMES IN LIFE when a new wardrobe is called for: not just regular updates to your clothes or for the fun of shopping, but transformations of one kind and another. A planned or real promotion, a maternity 'look', a post-baby revamp, a wardrobe to show off a lighter or tighter body, looking ahead to future decades, a shift in your life that you feel the need to reflect in your clothing: all of these are moments to plan a new wardrobe and your commute can be an enjoyable time to do this. Think about how you can use what you already have (or where and to whom existing clothes might be passed on to so that they are not wasted) and what you have always secretly wanted to own (go for it!). If you do some planning (e.g. about how many pairs of tops/bottoms etc. you'll actually need), chances are that you'll end up with a really great wardrobe that works for every occasion. Start your shopping list!

I have often said that I wish I had invented blue jeans: the most spectacular, the most practical, the most relaxed and nonchalant. They have expression, modesty, sex appeal, simplicity - all I hope for in my clothes.

Yves Saint Laurent

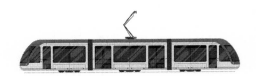

Nurture your soul

IT CAN BE GOOD SOMETIMES to stop our whirlwind of things to do, places to go, goals to hurry towards and instead to take a moment to be happy with what we already have, reach out to a stranger who may need a kind word or calm our racing minds. Use your commute to give your soul a chance to breathe and reach out to the fellow souls surrounding it on this voyage through life.

Life is short and we have never too much time for gladdening the hearts of those who are traveling the dark journey with us. Oh be swift to love, make haste to be kind.

Henri Frederic Amiel

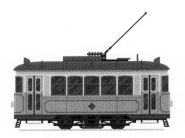

Travel with loved ones

WHEN I FIRST STARTED LIVING with my husband he used to leave for work about fifteen minutes earlier than I did. When I suggested that we should leave together (since we were heading to the same station) he looked appalled. "You walk too slowly," he complained. "Yes, but you get to work earlier than you need to anyway," I pointed out. So he left a little later and I left a little earlier so that we could go to work together and it didn't take long for him to agree that the commute was now improved: we had a ten minute walk holding hands and chatting together, followed by a companionable twenty minutes on the train together. We parted ways at a station along the route, giving us the chance for an extra kiss before heading off to our respective workplaces. Later on when we no longer traveled together, my husband would take our little boy to the childminder and pick him up again and he often said that picking him up and their ten minutes coming home together were one of the happiest parts of his day. Our neighbours have a similar arrangement where the dad takes his little girl with him to a crèche near his workplace and they enjoy their journeys together. You could even try and commute with friends or colleagues so that some of your journey time will pass in pleasant company.

I love to travel with my family or my two best friends because I completely trust them.

Julia Sawalha

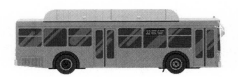

Smile at strangers

WHEN MY HUSBAND AND I walked to the station every day together, we regularly met two people. One was the street cleaner near our house, an older woman, originally from Ireland, who chatted and smiled at everyone who passed. We took to calling her 'Our Lady' as we didn't know her name, and looked out for her every day. She was so sunny and cheerful we missed her on the days when we didn't see her. She got to know us and if one of us came by without the other she would laugh and say, "Sure, you look like a lost sheep!" The other was a man who passed us every day walking in the opposite direction: we were going into central London and he worked somewhere locally. Because he looked like a younger version of the character nicknamed 'Horse' in the film *The Full Monty*, we called him Horse to ourselves. After we'd passed him for some months, I took to smiling at him in the mornings. The first day he looked a little startled but as we both started doing it he soon began to smile back at us every day. We never spoke, just smiled as we passed, but the day after terrorists bombed London, he stopped when he saw us and took our hands in his. "You take care," he said and we nodded, touched that we mattered to him. I'm sure you pass the same people every day. Smile at them and you'll come to matter to one another, even if you never know their name.

We shall never know all the good that
a simple smile can do.

Mother Teresa

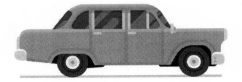

Make a difference

SEE IF YOU CAN DO one small kind thing every day on your way to or from work. You don't need to make grand gestures to make a difference. Help a parent struggling with a buggy, open a door for someone, allow another car to pull out in front of you with a cheerful wave instead of a grimace, offer a quick smile to let someone know it's okay that they trod on your foot by mistake and so on. See if you can make someone else's day easier, better or just a bit brighter. When it gets easy to do one thing, make it two things. And so on. If everyone was doing this all over the world... imagine the difference and get started.

I recently came across the notion of a 'blessing bag', to be given out to homeless people that you might see on your regular journey. You can make up your own but common items include: a bottle of water, juice, cereal bars, warm socks or gloves, dried fruit, savoury or sweet biscuits, baby wipes, toothbrush and toothpaste, toilet paper, hand sanitiser, a prepaid phone card or supermarket card and a note of encouragement and kindness.

You can also look out for people who may be having a bad day and try to say something to cheer them up. The famous #FindMike campaign showed what a big impact this can have when a passerby convinced a young man not to end his life by jumping off a bridge. The young man went on to build a happier life and had the opportunity to thank his Good Samaritan in person six years later.

On a smaller and more personal level, having one of those awful days that happen to everyone from time to time, struggling with a crying baby and feeling like a zombie from lack of sleep, I was hugely touched by an older lady who got off the train ahead of me and strode off, only to pause a good twenty yards away and come walking back to me as I tried to soothe my son. "You're very good with him – you look like a lovely mother," she said, and walked away again, leaving me in grateful tears at her kindness in taking a moment out of her own day to try and lift my spirits. I have never forgotten her. Look out for people who might need a kind word and don't be embarrassed to say something nice – people need it more than you might think.

My religion is very simple. My religion is kindness.

Dalai Lama

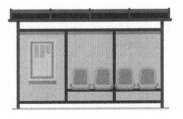

List your blessings

IT'S VERY EASY, ON A commute, to start mentally cataloguing everything that is wrong – no seat, too hot, all these annoying people, too much traffic – and for that to spiral off into everything you believe to be wrong in your life as a whole. Stop this kind of thinking before it gets depressing. Instead, take a deep breath and start listing the good things in your life. Start with the fundamental stuff: having enough to eat and drink, a roof over your head and take it from there. List tiny things (your electric toothbrush is freshly recharged and there's still toilet paper left in the cupboard) if that's all you can think of. You might even make yourself giggle and that's a good thing. If you can find big happy things such as a loving family and great friends, a good partner (even if they are annoying you right now this minute) and your health then keep going until you've listed them all. Go back into your past, look into your future and get as many good things as possible listed in your head (or even on a piece of paper if you need hard evidence). Feel your spirits lift as you focus on the good in your life. When you are feeling better, think of one thing that will improve whatever made you feel down in the first place. Just one. Don't get caught up in listing bad things or you'll be back at square one. Just find one small action that you can do very soon – sending your partner a loving text or booking an important appointment – that will improve the current situation. If you can do it on the commute, great. If you can't, do it as soon as you can. The more you focus on the good things, the less the smaller niggles will seem to matter and you will feel more positive.

Feel blessed in the life you have and make it better one tiny step at a time.

> Gratitude can transform common days into thanksgivings, turn routine jobs into joy, and change ordinary opportunities into blessings.
>
> William Arthur Ward

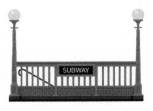

Read about good things

VARIOUS EXPERIMENTS HAVE BEEN DONE that show, for example, that if you read about being ill, you actually start behaving as though you *were* ill, while in another study, people who read about the Good Samaritan and were then put in a position where they had a chance to help someone, were far more likely to help than those who had not just read this parable. Try to read positive stories in the news and on the internet. Personally I dislike much of the news media because I think it takes a relentlessly negative attitude. I believe in looking at the positive in even the worse news stories. I think you will find that the world is actually mostly full of good people trying to achieve good things. Even in very bad situations, I challenge you to look and find who is doing something positive about it. Join in if you can: sign a petition, help out a charity, make sure bad things do not happen to those around you in whatever way you can. Read about people who are kind, talented and amazing. Read about great strides forward in improving planetary issues and look at the beautiful sights in the world, both natural and man-made. What you read changes you in subtle ways, so choose what you read with care. There are quite a few websites now devoted to telling good news stories and they make for seriously refreshing reading.

Melissa Addey

Most folks are as happy as they make
up their minds to be.

Abraham Lincoln

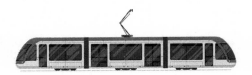

Plan time for relationships

Yes, you're stuck in traffic and your friends and family are not around. But you can use some of your commuting time to plan fun things to do together – whether it's popping round to see the neighbours or hosting a big party, a drive to visit family or inviting old friends out for a drink. Planning this time means you are more likely to focus on giving time to those relationships and enjoying time with those people who matter most to you. If you want to keep the flame burning with your partner, then a good idea is to spend some of your commuting time to plan something special for them. Perhaps a special outing, or a 'birthday book' with contributions from family and friends. I developed a list of 40 things for my husband to do for his 40th birthday. They will be touched by the fact that despite your busy life and having a lot of other plates to juggle you have still taken the time to think of their needs and what would make them happy. And you may find your thoughtfulness being reciprocated.

You can achieve all the things you want to do, but it's much better to do it with loved ones around you; family and friends, people that you care about that can help you on the way and can celebrate you, and you can enjoy the journey.

John Lasseter

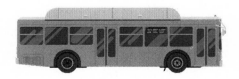

Send love to the kids

MY HUSBAND REGULARLY SETS OFF to work with one of our son's toy trains. Later, he'll send us a photo of the train on his desk, or at a meeting, which my son finds very funny indeed. On some apps (Whatsapp, Telegram, etc.) you can leave little voice recordings for the other person to play as a sort of audio version of a text. My son, as he can't yet write, enjoys recording these for his aunt and receiving them from her, asking to hear them over and over again. A whole day apart is a long time for small children and you may even be away for longer than that, so take a quick moment to create something fun or funny for them – they will love it.

Each day of our lives we make deposits
in the memory banks of our children.

Charles R. Swindoll

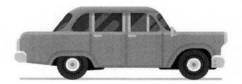

Practice Mindfulness

THIS IS A SIMPLE BUT very powerful exercise: simply be mindful of the moment you are in. Focus on everything your senses can offer you: the sounds around you and inside you, how your body feels, the movement of the vehicle as you travel, and so on. We forget to be present in our lives sometimes and even if you think you'd rather *not* be present, try this exercise anyway so that you accept the commute for what it is and stop railing against it.

With mindfulness, you can establish yourself in the present in order to touch the wonders of life that are available in that moment.

Nhat Hanh

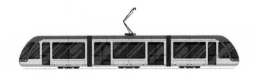

Take time to feel the love for your loved ones

TAKE A FEW MOMENTS TO think of the people you love in your life and enjoy the feeling, reminding yourself why you love them and that they love you. This is good on any day, but also if you've had an argument. It's also a good exercise to do if someone in your life is not all you'd like them to be – an annoying in-law or frustrating colleague. Think of them for a moment, don't focus on the bad but on the positive things about them, give them an interior smile and let any other feelings about them go. If you do this regularly you will bask in the love you have and improve other relationships around you a great deal.

Melissa Addey

I have no time for anything but trying to love other people. That is a full-time job.

Anne Rice

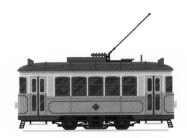

Meditate

D ON'T HAVE TIME TO ATTEND a meditation class or even for an at-home session all to yourself? Try and meditate during your commute – even just a brief session can be a calming and centring activity. If you are new to meditation but would like to give it a try, if only to escape the noise and motion around you and the stress you may be feeling, then just sit quietly and breathe. Notice your breath go in and out of you and let everything else go. If thoughts come up (as they will, of course: about what to make for dinner, about where you put your watch, about whether you remembered to do something) then just notice them and set them aside for later. You may feel silly at first or that you are not doing it 'right', but there is no right or wrong with this exercise, it is just a moment of stillness in your life - and we could all do with a few more of those. If you get interrupted, don't worry. Try again at the next available opportunity. You may find that this activity becomes a welcome and regular part of your commute.

.

Melissa Addey

Now I meditate twice a day for half an hour. In meditation, I can let go of everything. I'm not Hugh Jackman. I'm not a dad. I'm not a husband. I'm just dipping into that powerful source that creates everything. I take a little bath in it.

Hugh Jackman

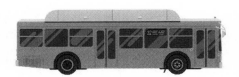

Stop and listen to the buskers

O N THE LONDON UNDERGROUND I'VE heard everything from opera to punk, rock to soul. And memorably, two people dressed as cats, who used to mime playing the saxophone, much to everyone's amusement. Some buskers are amazing and listening for a couple of minutes will not make you late. Enjoy the music and they will enjoy your attention. I once saw a couple dancing to a busker's waltz, which made everyone smile. Don't forget to drop a coin before you walk on! If you're in a car, try out a few different radio stations to get a taste of something different to your usual choices – you never know, you might stumble across a whole new musical love!

Where words fail, music speaks.

Hans Christian Andersen

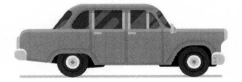

Pray

You might have a particular faith, in which case reading your holy book, reflecting on spiritual matters or praying may all be positive and uplifting things for you to do and ones with which you are familiar and find comforting. Some people read one page a day of a spiritual text, for example, or have a time when they take a moment to say a prayer. If you are not religiously inclined, you may still have an interest in matters spiritual and in this case you can develop your own spiritual progress or rituals and undertake them while you commute. You could even take this time to understand a little about other people's faiths and by doing so understand others better. Prayers do not need to be religious in nature if this is not for you, they can be simple expressions of hopes and fears, reflections and dreams. Try making a prayer you are happy with, whatever your beliefs, and say it or think it from time to time. Try it once even if you think this suggestion is not for you. You may surprise yourself.

I love you when you bow in your
mosque, kneel in your temple, pray in
your church. For you and I are sons of
one religion, and it is the spirit.

Khalil Gibran

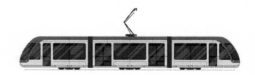

Find a new love

I F YOU ARE SINGLE AND searching for love, you can use your commute time as your very own quest for love. Start by actually identifying what you want from a relationship and then use dating sites, personal ads, let your friends know you'd like to be set up or even take a look around you! You might regularly spot someone on your commute that makes your heart beat a little faster. Work up the courage to ask them out. The worst they can say is no and you will probably make their day by asking even if they do turn you down — after all, everyone likes to be asked!

Romance is everything.

Gertrude Stein

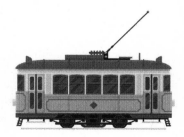

Laugh

WELL, YES, IT MIGHT BE embarrassing to be laughing out loud to yourself but actually I quite like seeing people laughing as they read a book on the train. I like that whatever they are reading is so funny it has overcome their natural inhibitions – and a person laughing is a happy sight anyway. Read or listen to funny books, listen to funny recordings such as comedians doing their shows, watch funny films. Starting and ending your working day laughing sounds good to me. If you're having a down day, make an effort to find something funny to enjoy and feel the difference it makes to your mood. Comedy shows have been fixing arguments between my husband and I for years: by the time you've laughed together at something for half an hour you've forgotten or forgiven what you were rowing about.

I like nonsense, it wakes up the brain cells. Fantasy is a necessary ingredient in living, it's a way of looking at life through the wrong end of a telescope. Which is what I do, and that enables you to laugh at life's realities.

Dr. Seuss

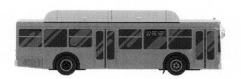

Keep in touch

You don't have to meet up with friends and family to be in touch with them. Social media means you can drop people a line any time and even a brief message or a 'like' means someone is thinking of you and is appreciated. Send your partner a text to make them smile, drop your friends a line on Facebook, call your mother, record a message for your little ones to hear. You could go old-style and keep a stack of funny or beautiful postcards and just send one off to friends and family from time to time. If you have time and won't bother others, put your phone on hands free and talk to friends and family. My postman at a previous address used to make me smile: he did all his rounds while happily chatting on his mobile's hands free kit: he must have been the best person at keeping in touch ever, as he spent several hours every day talking to the people in his life... or maybe just his fellow postmen! There are many ways to keep in touch and not all of them have to involve anything lengthy. My brother is not one for writing long letters or emails but he does love photo messages, so he'll regularly text me images of everything from the floor tiles in the house he is renovating to the family dog making a funny face. It's a little moment from his everyday life and I respond in kind with pictures of my children playing or the garden on a sunny day. Communication doesn't have to be about the big things, it can just be the tiny moments that make up your life and keep you in the loop with someone else's.

I have never let go of my childhood contacts. My best friends from childhood are still my best friends.

Oscar Hijuelos

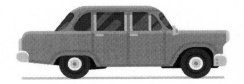

Indulge your passions

WHY NOT MAKE YOUR COMMUTE really special by focusing on your passions during it? Take your dreams and turn them into reality, indulge your hobbies or even turn your commute into a work of art. There are so many hobbies and passions, pursuits and pleasures out there and every person is different, so I won't have covered them all by any means but I hope the ideas listed here will give you an insight into how you can use your commute to do what makes you happiest. It's worth thinking about how you can develop a new passion or take your passion one step further, from watching films to making a documentary of your journey, from enjoying the theatre to joining an acting group and learning your lines as you travel.

To travel is to take a journey into yourself.

Danny Kaye

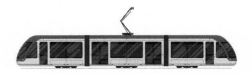

Enter a fantasy world

I USED TO REGULARLY SEE A man during my commute who was very into fantasy roleplay. He had books and magazines he would read, shielding them a little from other people's gaze as though he thought they were a bit embarrassing but I thought they looked quite interesting and would have liked to have known what sort of games he played (knowing nothing about this area of interest at all). I hope he managed to accumulate enough points to have the correct crystals, swords and magic potions at hand to make his commute a thrilling one!

I'm half living my life between reality and fantasy at all times.

Lady Gaga

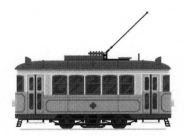

Spread the word

MY MOTHER'S FRIEND CARLO IS particularly fond of acting as a one-man PR machine for various causes of which he is fond. Speaking loudly into his switched off phone, he praises a friend's new book, suggests ways in which people might help out with a humanitarian crisis and encourages protest against badly-thought out government policies. He hopes, in his own small way, to pique the curiosity of those around him and spur them into action. Is there a cause that you can support through speaking on your phone to a non-existent friend? You never know who's listening.

Only one who devotes himself to a cause with his whole strength and soul can be a true master. For this reason mastery demands all of a person.

Albert Einstein

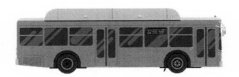

Run your own business

I T MAY BE THAT YOU have always secretly thought about running your own business but have not yet embarked on it, feeling perhaps that you don't have the time. But 1.5 hours per day means that you have 7.5 hours over the week – and that's one whole working day! So it could be a great opportunity to get started. Think about your business, write up a simple business plan – for yourself as much as anyone else, and take the first small steps. A lot of work can be outsourced, from logistics to manufacturing, and if you start small on your commute you'll be able to get a feel for whether your idea has legs before you commit to more time from your already busy life. You could also consider being a social entrepreneur, a growing area of business. And just think, if your business does take off, you'll be able to decide when and where you commute – if at all!

I've been an entrepreneur all my life, and my recent focus is on finding entrepreneurial solutions to address global challenges in healthcare and education.

Naveen Jain

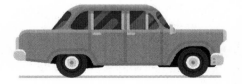

Write

M ANY PEOPLE HARBOUR A DESIRE to write and so here are a few ways to get started:

Do your Morning Pages. This is an exercise used by many writers and in particular recommended by Julia Cameron in her wonderful book, *The Artist's Way* (which lends itself very well to your commute as a 12-week series of writing exercises). You simply sit down every morning and write three pages. They may be drivel, they may be "I can't think what to write", written over and over again, they may be rants about the blocked kitchen sink or some other equally irritating small matter. It is a very useful exercise and worth doing even for just a few weeks to see what you think of it. Interesting things come and go when you do this exercise, from days when you feel it is a huge and tedious chore to days when you could write forever. If you are driving you might want to set yourself a target of talking out loud into a Dictaphone for five or ten minutes, just whatever comes into your head.

Write a novel. I recently read about a lawyer who wrote her first novel whilst commuting. If nothing else, at least write the first line. The Bulwer-Lytton competition awards a prize to the worst opening line of a novel, so you can amuse yourself by penning a *non*-masterpiece as a starting point. If you happen to come up with something that does actually sound good, then jot down some more thoughts around it and start that novel/short story/text book/ memoir you always meant to write. You could always enter the National Novel

Writing Month event, where your challenge is to knock out the first draft of a novel in one month. You can set yourself little writing challenges, such as writing about the journey, your fellow passengers and the funny little things you see every day which no-one else might notice. If you're driving, try dictating rather than writing – some novelists always write this way.

If a full-length novel sounds too daunting to start with then have a go at flash fiction and short stories: there are lots of competitions to enter if you do, which can be fun. These shorter forms can lend themselves nicely to a commute.

> Every story I create, creates me. I write to create myself.
>
> Octavia E. Butler

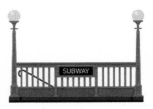

Let out your inner poet

POETRY CAN BE A LOVELY thing to read while on your commute. Or try writing some poetry yourself. No, it doesn't have to rhyme! Try limericks, haiku and micro poetry or just dive right in there and get on with your odes, epics and pastorals. The Poetry Foundation's website has a great page listing all the different forms of poetry, which makes for an interesting read in itself and you might just find some forms that suit you. Found poetry, for example, could be perfect for the commute, when you bring together unconnected words and phrases seen around you, even within boring work reports.

Poetry is when an emotion has found
its thought and the thought has found
words.

Robert Frost

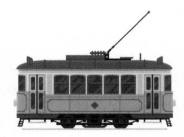

Enter stage left

I T'S FAIR TO SAY THAT it's unlikely you'll find Shakespeare being performed in your train carriage or on your bus. But if you love theatre then you can find ways to bring it into your commute. Book tickets for plays, read plays, watch recordings of plays, listen to plays on the radio or as downloads, read up on actors, playwrights and particular productions. Write your own play! If you're part of an acting group or class then your commute is a great time to learn your lines.

I think there is no world without theatre.

Edward Bond

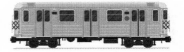

Make friends at work

Most people at your workplace will be commuting too, and having good friends at work can be a very positive part of your worklife. Developing friendships can often be helped along by shared experiences, so why not suggest that all of you who commute get set little challenges – such as bringing in a new foodstuff to try as a team or finding the weirdest advert in your carriage? Snap a picture and bring it in, give out little prizes once a week for fun and see if your team grows closer as a result.

When we asked people if they would rather have a best friend at work or a 10% pay raise, having a friend clearly won.

Tom Rath

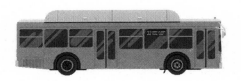

Become an all-out foodie

I F YOU LOVE FOOD THEN use your commute to plan new menus, find new recipes, read up on restaurants and book a table, order a new cookbook, arrange foodie events like supper clubs and even order your food shopping for the week. Join a chocolate tasting club where you get sent a box of chocolates every month, then take one with you each day to sweeten your journey.

What I've enjoyed most, though, is meeting people who have a real interest in food and sharing ideas with them. Good food is a global thing and I find that there is always something new and amazing to learn – I love it!

Jamie Oliver

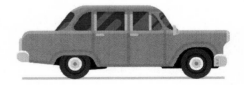

Play computer games

F IND A GAME TO PLAY, from board games to video games. *Solitaire, Candy Crush, Angry Birds... Call of Duty* or whatever is your new favourite. If you want to go all Grand Master about it you can also play things like chess and Scrabble with people online, since you can do one move at a time and come back when they've made their move. You can rediscover old favourites from your childhood or try out the latest game everyone's been going on about. This idea does not, however, work quite as well if you are inclined to get in a rage because you can't manage to knock things down satisfactorily, shoot up enough zombies or your winning score is not your personal best. If that's the case, perhaps you'd be better off with the meditation suggestion I made earlier. Alternatively, start studying the rules of bridge, poker and other card games and improving your game. Maybe Las Vegas won't know what's hit it!

While films are a very visual and emotional artistic medium, video games take it one step further into the realm of a unique personal experience.

Jet Li

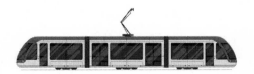

Develop your artistic nature

DRAWING AND PAINTING CAN BE great on a commute. Draw what's around you or something from your imagination, practice some aspect of the craft that you've never quite managed to get right or simply enjoy playing with light and shadow, different colours and ideas. If you feel that you can't draw at all then challenge yourself to have a go: steal your child's crayons for a little while, get some paper and see what emerges. We all need a bit of playtime. There's some great photos on the Pinterest board for this book of a guy who draws cartoon heads for his fellow commuters. If creating art isn't for you but you love art anyway then enjoy great works of art in books or on your phone or laptop and book yourself a ticket to the latest exhibition.

Colour is my day-long obsession, joy
and torment.

Claude Monet

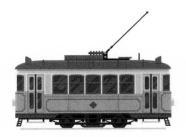

Get crafty

THERE ARE ALL KINDS OF crafts you can do while you commute – woodwork (on a small scale!), embroidery, knitting, spinning, cross-stitch, sewing, papercraft, jewellery and more. If your craft is larger-scale, like restoring or refurbishing furniture, then you can be reading books about techniques and planning new styles while you travel. If you're a beginner but like the sound of some of these crafts then there are lots of starter kits and books available so that you can begin your craft journey while you travel.

We are all apprentices in a craft
where no one ever becomes a master.

Ernest Hemingway

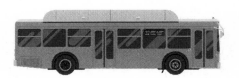

Change your mood with music.

MUSIC CAN CHANGE YOUR MOOD quite radically. It can cheer you up, it can calm you down and it can give you back your energy on an exhausting day. I suggest you make up a playlist of your favourite music – or even multiple ones for different mood shifts as required. Your favourite piece of music can usually make you smile, so know what it is and have it to hand so you can change the day's tempo. Shake up your musical ruts by asking for new music as a gift or tune in to a different radio station. If you need to be quiet, then you can learn sheet music or lyrics. If you can be loud, then sing! You can get vocal exercises to follow if you'd like to make your voice stronger and lovelier – and these exercises are good for presentations and speeches as well as singing. Read up on your favourite artists and order their new albums.

Music drives you. It wakes you up, it gets you pumping. And, at the end of the day, the correct tune will chill you down.

Dimebag Darrell

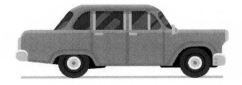

Use your camera

G ET CREATIVE WITH YOUR CAMERA or even with your phone's camera. Look out for interesting things to photograph during your commute and set yourself little challenges or themes to develop over time. There are some nice photography books that set you such challenges for a whole year. If you're an amateur then now's the time to read the camera manual or at least play with the different settings so you work out what they actually do. You may end up with panoramic vistas of people's feet, but that's still fun. If you're driving then perhaps spot good new opportunities for photography that you can return to at a later date or pull over once a day and take a photo. If you take the time to play, you'll be a better photographer after just a few commuting sessions, as you'll find out what works and what doesn't and why rather than pressing the button and hoping for the best. Use Pinterest and Instagram to share meaningful images, create and order a photo book online, edit your own photos and use Instagram or other sites to follow great photographers so that you can sit and scroll through your very own photography exhibition.

Whoever controls the media, the images, controls the culture.

Allen Ginsberg

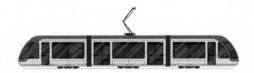

Release the fashionista in you

I F YOU LOVE FASHION AND all things clothing related then use your commute to read your favourite fashion magazines, style blogs and books, plan a new wardrobe of clothes, do online window shopping, collect images of clothes you desperately want, make your own clothes while you travel, sell your unwanted treasures online and bid for others. If you're not in a hurry you can get great bargains on eBay and outlet sites for your favourite brands as you will know what size you are. Swap tips with other fashion fanatics online and plan shopping trips. Figure out your own personal style.

Fashion fades, only style remains the same.

Coco Chanel

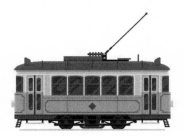

Redesign your home

Y OU MAY LOVE INTERIOR DESIGN or have taken on a real
project of a house that needs serious renovation. Whether
you need some pretty cushions or a total re-wiring, use your
commute time to plan what needs doing, source materials and
tradesmen, compare paint colours and shop online for items
you need. A lot of design and renovation is actually about the
thinking – understanding what the real purpose of a room is
or how you can make the most of what you've already got,
so use your commute time to think carefully so that when it
comes to the action part, you won't make (too many) mistakes.

There is no society ever discovered
in the remotest corner of the world
that has not had something that we
would consider the arts. Visual arts
- decoration of surfaces and bodies -
appears to be a human universal.

Steven Pinker

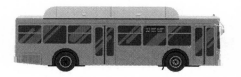

Be entranced by the silver screen

Y OUR COMMUTE IS A GREAT time to catch up on all the films you meant to see but never quite got round to. Get a good subscription service and you'll be away. See some old classics, catch up on your favourite film stars' careers or go all out and create themed seasons to get through. If you want to get even more immersed, make your own films: from stop-motion animation to filming your commute as though it were a documentary. Even pretty basic phones come with a video camera, so have some fun with it.

Perhaps I am old-fashioned, but black and white films still hold an affectionate place in my heart; they have an incomparable mystique and mood.

Ginger Rogers

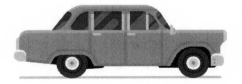

Read books

YOUR COMMUTE GIVES YOU A lot of reading time! Make a list of books you'd love to read or ask people you know for recommendations and get going. Try novels, self-help, interesting how-to books and books that explore all sorts of new subjects or topics that you have a particular interest in. If you have an e-reader there are often a lot of promotional deals going so you can fill up your device with good value reads. Your local library is also worth a visit to see what they have that interests you, while charity shops usually have a lot of cheaply priced books available. My local train station actually has a book swap bookcase available – you can grab any book you want and return it or bring in something new to swap with it – it's been going a few years now and I think it's a great idea. Remember audio books, too: there are thousands available so whatever book you'd like to read there's probably an audio book of it available.

Once you've really gotten the bookworm bug then perhaps you'd like to be part of a bookclub with friends or colleagues. I belong to a bookclub made up of five friends, which has now been going for ten years. Because we live all over town, we usually meet somewhere central once a month, have a nice meal together and discuss the book, as well as many other things along the way. If setting one up feels like too much of a commitment right now, you might want to join one online: there are bookclubs on the radio as well as in some newspapers such as *The Guardian*. Much of the work is done for you: a book will be chosen, it is discussed by experts and you the reader can read along and add your comments to the accompanying blog or just read other people's thoughts. It's a nice way to explore a book in more depth than you might usually do and feel part of a wider community of readers. Also, if you are part of a bookclub and accept each book that is chosen, you get to read titles you would never have selected yourself, and this can be very interesting, since everyone tends to get stuck in genre ruts from time to time.

> I know that books seem like the ultimate thing that's made by one person, but that's not true. Every reading of a book is a collaboration between the reader and the writer who are making the story up together.
>
> John Green

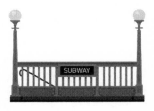

Plan your green space

ALRIGHT, SO YOU CAN'T START digging up the road but you can certainly plan your green space, be it garden, balcony or just house plants. Order seeds and plants, do an online garden design course or read gardening books. You could even volunteer to look after the plants at your local train station as you pass by. If you want to feel adventurous, try guerrilla gardening, where you throw seed 'bombs' (balls of dried mud embedded with flower seeds) onto unused patches of land that you pass and have the pleasure of watching flowers bloom on barren soil. One community completely changed a bus stop like this and one town did so much of this that they ended up with free patches of herbs such as rosemary and sage that anyone passing by could take home to cook with.

Flowers always make people better, happier, and more helpful; they are sunshine, food and medicine for the soul.

Luther Burbank

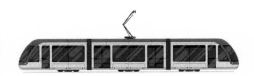

Travel

I F YOU ARE AN INTREPID traveler then the boring back and forth of your commute may feel frustrating. Plan and book your next holiday, read travel books and travelogues, learn a bit of the language for your next destination, order holiday essentials, swap travel tips online and even pen a travel book yourself – or contribute to famous titles such as the Lonely Planet series, which will list you in their next edition if you send them hints, tips and feedback for one of their destinations.

Perhaps travel cannot prevent bigotry, but by demonstrating that all peoples cry, laugh, eat, worry, and die, it can introduce the idea that if we try and understand each other, we may even become friends.

Maya Angelou

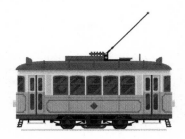

Follow your dreams

M Y DREAM WAS TO BE a full-time writer. I sort of am now, although it's alongside being a mother so guess how much time I get to write?! While my first child napped, I wrote a novel. With my second baby, as I breastfed, I wrote the notes that made up a parenting book. I proofed this book while commuting. I grabbed every chance I got to move closer to my dream of being a writer. So what would you like to do? What is your big dream? And would an hour and a half or more every day be of use to you in moving closer to that dream? I'm pretty sure it would. Take some time to focus on what your dreams and goals are and then use your commute to get one tiny step closer to them. It doesn't matter if it's just a little move forwards, it's a move all the same and you might be surprised at what it leads on to. Also, it's a funny thing, but often once you've focused on a goal, opportunities seem to present themselves to help you move towards achieving it, perhaps simply because you notice them more. So sit and daydream for a while, then identify your own dreams and think of what you can do while commuting to make them happen. And commit your dream to paper. It makes a difference.

All our dreams can come true, if we
have the courage to pursue them.

Walt Disney

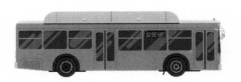

Head for the great outdoors

WELL, RIGHT NOW YOU'RE SORT of stuck inside some means of transport, but you can be planning for outdoor pursuits if they are your passion. From sports to camping, fishing to skydiving, use your commute to plan outings, read up on techniques, purchase items you need, find similarly-enthusiastic friends, family and online acquaintances to share your events with and read the adventures of others who share your passions. Watch sports events or replays, share comments on the online forums, listen to radio commentary, book tickets to or seek out older films that feature your outdoor loves from hiking to mountain climbing, flying to fishing. At least by the time your commute is over you'll have made plans and be all fired up for your next adventure.

Melissa Addey

If you drive to, say, Shenandoah National Park, or the Great Smoky Mountains, you'll get some appreciation for the scale and beauty of the outdoors. When you walk into it, then you see it in a completely different way. You discover it in a much slower, more majestic sort of way.

Bill Bryson

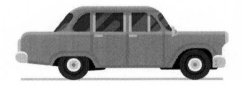

Bring animals into your life

You may be a great lover of animals in which case you could make some time for them and find ways to bring them into your life while you travel. Take your dog to work if your employer allows it, some workplaces find that a pet becomes a mascot for the whole team. Read up on a pet you'd like to own so you choose a suitable animal for your lifestyle. Read up on training tips if you get a dog so that you treat it appropriately and have a pet that is manageable in all situations. Offer to help out with animal charities, book a horse riding lesson, find and buy a new pet from a reputable source (if you can support an animal shelter, so much the better) or even sponsor an animal if you can't keep a pet – perhaps something you'd love to own in real life. Plan trips to zoos, city farms and safaris or book a holiday on a working farm.

The greatness of a nation can be judged by the way its animals are treated.

Mahatma Gandhi

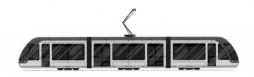

Do something charitable

YOU MAY ALREADY BE INVOLVED in charitable work or have always wanted to do something for others. There are some things you can start to do on your commute: sign petitions online, buy charitable gifts or make donations, arrange charity events and sign yourself up for a charity run or walk. Take some donations along with you and drop them off somewhere along your commute, give out 'blessing bags' to the homeless people you pass each day, find a charity you could volunteer for and sign up with them, order bags from charities for your home and office so that you can send off used ink cartridges to be recycled, which gives many charities a small donation. Write a letter to a prisoner or other person in need, sponsor a child (to whom you can also write letters) or even just go to one of the many online sites to 'click' and thereby encourage donations to many charitable efforts. Also think about those closer to you and see if you can find a way to help them out – join the local Neighborhood Watch scheme, invite an old neighbour around for a cup of coffee or offer to help out at a local school.

Where there is charity and wisdom,
there is neither fear nor ignorance.

Francis of Assisi

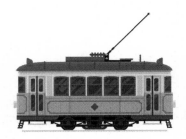

Advance your career

S INCE YOU'RE TRAVELING TO WORK you might want to consider spending some of your commute on your career. Let me be clear though, I think spending your commute answering work emails, drafting work reports, etc. is a massive waste of your own personal time. However, there can be some benefits to doing some work-related activities, if they are going to be of personal benefit to you. Here are some ideas.

How often I found where I should be going only by setting out for somewhere else.

R. Buckminster Fuller

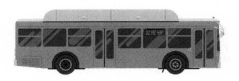

Be in the know

I F YOU ARE KEEN ON your industry and job then it is worth spending a bit of time on your commute keeping up to date with your industry's news, trends and future. Get a subscription to a suitable trade journal (your work will often pay for this) and become a fountain of knowledge about your own industry. People are often so busy with their day-to-day role that they don't bother to look around and keep up to date, let alone look to the future, and they can be caught unawares as a result. You will do better at your job and look impressive to your employer if you are industry-savvy.

Never become so much of an expert
that you stop gaining expertise.
View life as a continuous learning
experience.

Denis Waitley

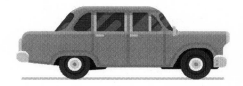

Get in early, stay late

I ACTUALLY HATE WORKPLACES WHERE IT becomes a habit or culture that people must get in early or stay late every day just to be seen doing so. Are they paying you for that time? I don't think so. I've been in one too many offices where people are still at their desks as I walk out of the door – and I can see that all they are doing is playing Solitaire on their PC. Please. Having said that, there is a case to be made for occasionally coming in early or staying late – apart from the obvious that your commute will probably be quieter. It may be that your boss is hard to get a word with but that if you're in early on a Thursday you can catch them for a cup of coffee and get to know them and their needs better and let them know what a good job you're doing. Worth the extra time. Or if you stay late on a Tuesday there's networking drinks with a department where you need to build better links. Might be useful. Please don't get caught up in doing this all the time, just pick and choose when and where it can help you out.

Early to bed and early to rise makes a
man healthy, wealthy and wise.

Benjamin Franklin

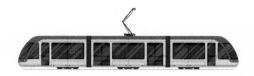

Get better qualified

I S THERE A QUALIFICATION THAT you know you need or that would really improve your promotional and career opportunities? Then I'd suggest your commute would be a great place to start working on it. Your workplace may well be inclined to pay for it and if you can use your commuting time then getting that qualification need not eat into your private life too much. I took a Postgraduate Certificate over the course of a year in my job, which was beneficial to my career and I did most of the reading for it on my commute.

Education is the key to unlock the golden door of freedom.

George Washington Carver

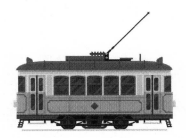

Have a special project

I SPENT A FEW OF MY lunch hours at work developing a report. I hadn't been asked to do it, but it showed the social benefit of my organisation's work (which was usually measured only in commercial terms). It was quite interesting to write anyway, but when I showed it to my boss he was very impressed and showed it to a director, who then showed it to the Board. The end result for me was that I got put onto the bid-writing team, which I had wanted to get onto for some time. That report didn't take a lot of my personal time but it did move me into a place where I could learn some new skills that mattered to me. Is there a project you can develop and work on during your commute that will shine a spotlight on you and take you to new places in your career?

The biggest mistake that you can make is to believe that you are working for somebody else. Job security is gone. The driving force of a career must come from the individual. Remember: Jobs are owned by the company, you own your career!

Earl Nightingale

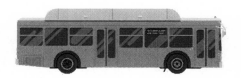

Make a career plan

D O YOU HAVE A CAREER plan? Most people don't, so give yourself an advantage by spending some time working out what you want to do next and how to get there. Do you need to get a new qualification? Upgrade your wardrobe? Spend more time socialising with the boss or within different social circles? Be willing to travel? Take on a special project to stand out from the crowd? Go on secondment to learn new skills? Think about this year, next year, and five years' time away for starters. Where you'd like to be, how to get there and what you can do right now to get closer to your goals. Maybe after all that career planning you can plan a sabbatical too!

When I was 14 years old, I made this PowerPoint presentation, and I invited my parents into my room and gave them popcorn. It was called 'Project Hollywood 2004' and it worked. I moved to L.A. in January of 2004.

Emma Stone

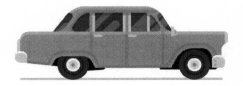

Work smarter

TAKE A BIT OF TIME to figure out how to work smarter rather than harder. Get a good book on time management and while you commute do some work on better diary management, delegation, automating some of your work (e.g. automatic email sorting) and so on. Find good people you can team up with to work better together. If you can work smarter you'll take away some of the tedious stuff and be able to spend more time on the parts of your job you really enjoy.

I'm smart enough to know to work with smart people.

Idina Menzel

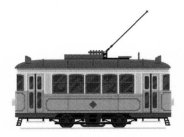

Get paid more

MANY PEOPLE CAN FEEL AWKWARD about asking for a pay rise, but preparation is the key to success in this quest and you can spend a bit of your commuting time to make sure that you put together a convincing case for a pay rise, such as listing accomplishments and praise, new responsibilities you've taken on and checking other jobs in the marketplace to make sure you know what you're worth.

I think the girl who is able to earn her own living and pay her own way should be as happy as anybody on earth. The sense of independence and security is very sweet.

Susan B. Anthony

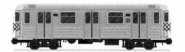

Find a new job

I F YOU'RE NOT ACTUALLY THAT keen on your current job, the pay rise has been turned down or your career plan has shown you a need for change, then there's always the option to change jobs. Realistically, few of us want to job search in work time as it sort of gives the game away, and you may be busy at home, so take advantage of your commute to identify the work you'd really like to do with the use of a good book like *How to Get a Job You'll Love* by John Lees, set up job email alerts (to your home email address, please!), read up on the marketplace, get yourself put on headhunter and agency lists, update your CV, identify new qualifications you might need, do some online window shopping for a smart interview suit or fill in interminable job application forms – and then, of course, practice your interview questions. Good luck!

Whether you're scared of getting into a relationship; or taking the new job; or a confrontation - you have to size fear up.

Chris Pine

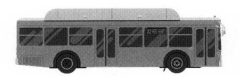

Free up your free time

Y ES, YOUR COMMUTE SHOULD BE a happy and interesting time for you. But the reality is that you are constrained in some ways: physically there's only so much you can do and your employer will expect to see you turn up at some point, at least on your way into work! A lot of commuters complain that their commute takes up a lot of their personal time, meaning when they get home there are still chores to be done and their 'free' time isn't quite as free as they'd like. So one approach is to use your commute as a useful 'chores' time, so that when you do get home, you are free to do something more fun.

Melissa Addey

The use of traveling is to regulate imagination by reality, and instead of thinking how things may be, to see them as they are.

Samuel Johnson

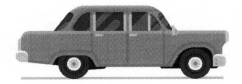

Keep up with correspondence

E MAILS STACK UP WHEN WE'RE busy and a full inbox can be a stressful and depressing sight. They may be personal or work related, but take a little time each day to clear down as many as you can – answer the easy ones quickly, sort out any small tasks that you were supposed to do (putting dates in calendars, answering invitations, booking the dentist, etc.) so that you can get rid of those too and then try to deal with one or two harder ones – more complex issues, longer replies required and so on. Take the opportunity to unsubscribe from anything you no longer want to receive, as this usually needs doing every couple of months anyway. Send out the odd few photos of your life to family and friends rather than long-winded accounts of how you are, it's quicker and more fun. If you can't give a proper answer to something then send a holding email to say you'll get back to someone so that at least you don't feel hounded or guilty. Get used to using online services for invitations, scheduling meet-ups (Doodle is the best thing ever for organising group meetings!) and if you're behind on your birthday greetings then use a card or gift service. Order pre-printed Christmas cards so that you can write personal messages rather than all the repetitive bits.

I long to accomplish a great and noble task, but it is my chief duty to accomplish small tasks as if they were great and noble.

Helen Keller

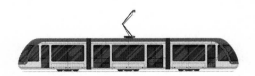

Write to-do lists

I AM AN INVETERATE LIST-MAKER, SO I always have a notepad somewhere nearby with long lists of things to do scribbled all over its pages. Some get done, others don't, but writing things down can mean that you are reminded of their importance as well as getting the satisfaction of crossing them off when they're done. It also means letting go of them from inside your brain, so that you don't spend time worrying about them. Your to-do list can be everything from the day-to-day stuff to the more adventurous: from changing the cat litter to ideas for a great holiday, but chances are if it's written down it'll get done. If some of the tasks on the list are massive and daunting then see if you can break them down into bite-sized pieces. It's also quite satisfying to make a to-do list for each year of your main goals, break them down into the small bits and watch as the list slowly gets ticked off as the year goes by!

Melissa Addey

My to-do list is so long that it doesn't
have an end; it has an event horizon.

Craig Bruce

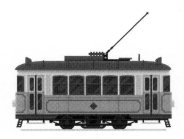

Get the shopping done

Don't waste your weekend traipsing round supermarkets doing the same old grocery shopping. Most supermarkets will now deliver your order to your home, so I am a big fan of online shopping. Do your weekly shop online while you commute, book a convenient slot for the shopping's arrival, then sit back and wait. Because most people's weekly shop is pretty similar week in week out, your supermarket usually keeps your favorite items as a ready-made list, meaning you can do your shopping in about 20 minutes online. No heavy bags to carry, no driving (or struggling with said bags on public transport), just your shopping delivered to your door.

If this is already familiar to you then consider shopping for most other things online too. Even if you like to support small companies, most businesses do online shopping. You can browse for what you need, order it online and have it delivered to your door – my little boy loves all the parcels we get and I love not having to drag him round the shops for things we need. When my baby was born just before Christmas, all my holiday food, Christmas cards, even gifts, were bought and dispatched online – there are companies that can pre-print your cards and many will gift-wrap your gifts and send them directly to the recipient. Makes your life a lot easier and it will free up time to do other things that can't be so easily done while commuting (game of tennis, anyone?).

Melissa Addey

I went window-shopping today! I
bought four windows.

Tommy Cooper

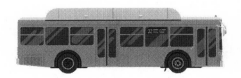

Plan and research all that stuff that needs doing

A LOT OF STUFF IN LIFE needs planning or research. Holidays, house-hunting if you're looking for a new home, finding someone to car share with, finding childcare or schools for your children are all good things to do while you commute. You can also book appointments like the dentist, doctor, hairdresser or plan social events with friends. Anything that needs planning, research and booking is good material to work on while you commute. Use this time wisely and you'll find yourself getting more done that you'd believe possible.

One big thing you can do, especially if you have kids, is plan your meals for the week. Standing in front of cupboards and fridges pondering what to make for each meal gets boring and doesn't really inspire creative solutions. Making a meal planner for the week means your shopping will be more efficiently tailored to what you are actually going to use and means you will always know what you're supposed to be cooking (you can switch meals round if you don't fancy what's on the menu that day!). I have a blank one-page sheet with a table that contains the date/days of the week and Breakfast/Lunch/Supper for each as well as space for notes, e.g. someone coming to lunch. I fill it in once a week and then do the shopping. The list then gets stuck up in the kitchen and solves meal dilemmas for the rest of the week. At the bottom, we scribble things we've run out of for next week's shop. It saves a lot of time and energy as well as allowing us to plan ahead and introduce interesting new meals to try on appropriate days like the weekends when everyone has a bit more time for experimenting. Make your own little sheet and use the time while commuting to create your menu for the week: you'll have nicer food and spend less time worrying about what to make

Each minute is a little thing, and yet, with respect to our personal productivity, to manage the minute is the secret of success.

Joseph B. Wirthlin

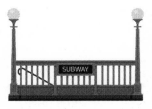

Update your technology

THERE'S SO MANY SILLY LITTLE things we forget to do or don't bother to do and then get annoyed because we put them off and now we need them. Now is the time to say "yes" when your computer asks if it can update your software. It's the time to install and programme new software and apps that can do everything from satellite navigation (no more getting lost or rows in the car over map-reading) to planning meetings and social occasions, set up live bus arrival times for your local bus stops, diary reminder entries for everyone's birthdays and arrange text alerts from your bank before you go overdrawn. It's the time to find a game that will entertain your toddler and download it to your phone and the time to update your contact lists and address book. Or just have fun 'training' your voice recognition software. These are the boring little things we never get round to but then wish we had because they make our lives smoother, quicker and better informed. Sort out these little bits, you'll be glad of them later.

One machine can do the work of fifty ordinary men. No machine can do the work of one extraordinary man.

Elbert Hubbard

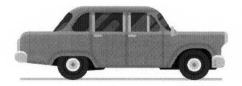

Do your work prep

I've said before that I'm not a big fan of working outside your normal hours because I think your commute time is your time, not work time. Having said that, sometimes it can be good to be ahead of the game and if you have to catch up then your commute can be a good time to do so. Read company reports, prepare mentally for a presentation, grade papers, prepare for your annual appraisal. Make the most of this time to get the boring work things done and dusted so that when you reach home you are free to get on with your personal life again.

The best preparation for good work
tomorrow is to do good work today.

Elbert Hubbard

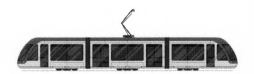

Get to grips with your paperwork

W HEN'S THE LAST TIME YOU actually looked at your bank statement properly? Take this time to sit and look through it in detail. You'll notice anything untoward more quickly if it happens (e.g. people fraudulently using your cards), realise bad spending habits - my husband pointed out that little 'top-up' shops at the supermarket were adding up to a few hundred in cash a year - and avoid bank charges like overdraft usage if you make a few changes to how you manage your money. Also take a moment to check on things like the list of direct debits you have and cancel any that are no longer of benefit, like gym memberships you don't use or magazines you are no longer interested in. You'll be surprised how poring over a boring piece of paper can reap real financial rewards from time to time. Take a look at comparison sites online and see if you are paying over the odds for utilities and make the switch. Sort out important paperwork like making a will or getting life insurance — you usually have to request quotes and fill in some forms so you can start scribbling your basic answers while travelling.

Melissa Addey

Getting paperwork under control
makes me feel more in control of my
life generally.

Gretchen Rubin

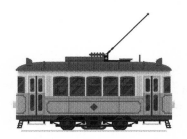

Sort out your photos

WE'RE TAKING MORE PHOTOS THAN ever because we have cameras built into our phones and our cameras are digital so we don't feel like we are using up expensive film. But do these photos ever get seen again? This can be a good time to sort them into files and choose ones to print. You can then upload them to photo sites (I've used various including Photo Box) where they will be printed and posted back to you in a matter of days. Many sites also now make really nice printed photo albums which can record holidays, babies, weddings, family recipes and more. I made one for my first baby and am currently making a family cookbook: again, find a photo site, upload the photos you want to use, have fun arranging them in a book (there are lots of different layouts to choose from) and then sit back and wait for a lovely professional-looking album to drop through your letterbox.

To me, photography is an art of observation. It's about finding something interesting in an ordinary place... I've found it has little to do with the things you see and everything to do with the way you see them.

Elliott Erwitt

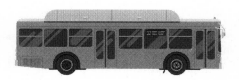

Declutter (mentally)

YOU MIGHT THINK THAT DECLUTTERING your house or life is going to involve standing there putting things into boxes to take to a charity shop or the recycling bin. Which is true, but most decluttering happens in your head first. Imagine the areas you need to declutter and think about what has to go. You can do this with your clothes, books, kids' toys, music and more. Just spend some time thinking about what needs to go and then when it comes to the actual action of sorting it out, it will take a lot less time because you will have already have identified what needs to go. You can also shop for better storage online if this is part of the problem.

One way to organise your thoughts is to tidy up, even if it's in places where it makes no sense at all.

Ursus Wehrli

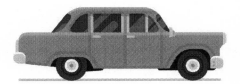

Change your commute altogether

S O: YOU'VE IMPLEMENTED PLENTY OF my suggestions and your commute has become a little happier but you still don't really *enjoy* it. Maybe it's time to change it altogether, so here are some ideas to help you with that. Again, remember that it is *your* commute and you can choose to change it for the better – but there may well be a tradeoff. Think about what matters most to you and what you are willing to give up as well as what you will get out of a big change to your commute.

If you want to succeed you should strike out on new paths, rather than travel the worn paths of accepted success.

John D. Rockefeller

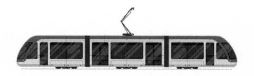

Move house

U NLESS YOU ARE LIVING IN the house of your dreams, then consider moving closer to work. Imagine living a five-minute walk from your job. Your commute would be amazing. Impossible? Not always. It depends where you are willing to live and how much space you need. Even if your commute was only a twenty-minute walk, wouldn't that be great? If you are serious about this idea, then get a map showing your worplace. Draw a circle around it that is the distance you'd be happy with commuting within and now you have the reality of a move in front of you. Is it possible? If you love your work and hate your commute and where you live is negotiable, then start negotiating. This tip will probably work best for younger commuters who perhaps need less space than commuters with families who need more space, but everyone should take a moment to consider it as a possibility.

By the way, if you *are* in the house of your dreams, then remember that you chose to live there and you also chose where to work, so your commute is something you chose. At the time, you must have thought it was acceptable. What's changed? When you've figured that out, you'll know what to do to make it better.

I love moving. I love new houses. I'm always looking for somewhere else.

Elizabeth Hurley

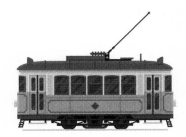

Move job

No, DON'T *LEAVE* (THAT'S NEXT on the list). Move. It's possible that you work for a large company that has more than one location. Can you apply to be transferred? Look into this. Be warned that it may take some time: a friend waited almost a year but then got the transfer he wanted so he could set up home with his girlfriend in a place that suited both of them. Conversely, if you work for a really tiny company, do you get any say in where you are based? I worked for a small company and head office was really only where it was because the owner of the company lived nearby. We had one additional rented office in the centre of town and when the lease came up on it we got a say in where the office should be based. Workplaces that are less centrally based (e.g. if you don't need to see clients) may also cost less so you might be doing your boss a favour by suggesting a new location if the opportunity arises.

It used to be presumed that if you weren't at your desk working, you weren't working. But we said, "Why can't we make a workplace where casual meetings are as important as working at your desk?" Sometimes that's where your better creative work happens.

David Chipperfield

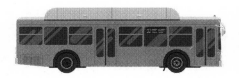

Change job

WELL IF YOU'RE NOT GOING to move house and your workplace isn't going to move... then have you thought about changing your job? This obviously is one for the people who don't much like their jobs and are already looking elsewhere, but it's an important thing to bear in mind when you are looking for a new place. If you've hated your commute for a long time, make it a priority to improve matters in your next job: look for jobs closer to home or with better transport links, perhaps jobs that are based somewhere where your commute will take you against the normal traffic flow so that your journey may be just as long but more relaxing or comfortable. Also look for jobs that are more flexible in *how* you work (see the next two points).

I still get the jitters every time I start
a new job! I love it - makes you feel
alive.

Camille Guaty

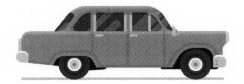

Change how often you commute

S O RIGHT NOW YOU GET up and go to work and come home again. Twice a day, every day, you make the same journey. So perhaps it's time to shake things up a little, if your work will consider a request for more flexible working.

First of all, if you are in your dream home but a long way from work, consider staying overnight. There are people who have a nice house somewhere outside the city and perhaps a cheap room in a shared apartment somewhere close to work. They come into work on Monday, go home on Friday. This may or may not work, depending on the hours you work and how your family would feel about you being absent during the week, but it is an option. You will save money on commuting, which can go towards the rent; and many people would be glad to share an apartment with someone who is not there at the weekend.

The next option is to work from home one or more days a week. I was hugely lucky to work for a company which allowed all of our team to work from home, all week. We had work mobile phones, we had laptops that connected to the work servers and we occasionally attended team meetings in a central location, which was hired by the hour. The company saved a lot of money on renting an office and we were all very happy with the freedom from the daily commute. Yes, you have to be disciplined to work from home but in my view the discipline was worth the freedom a hundred times over. I had three hours a day in my own house to myself (2 commuting hours and my lunch break) so I could get a lot done (household chores, my own projects, time with my family) and I felt good about being trusted to manage my own time and workload. It worked really well for me and on the day when there was a major snowfall and no-one went to work, our team were all still working, so there were some unexpected perks for the employers, too! My husband works from home one day a week. We benefit as a family from more time together on that day and he avoids the commute. I sometimes get to go out to socialize with my friends a little earlier that day as I don't have to wait an extra hour for him to arrive home but can leave when he finishes work. His work also benefits as this is a good day for him to tackle big projects that could do with no interruptions, such as writing complex reports or planning long-term strategic work.

A final option is to work your usual hours but in less time. Could you do 5 days' worth of work in 4 days? Some people prefer to do this kind of pattern. Think about your work and discuss options with your employer. You might be surprised at what they are willing to consider.

Don't wait. The time will never be just right.

Napoleon Hill

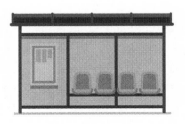

Change when you commute

A DIFFERENT WAY TO ALTER YOUR commute is to think about what makes the commute hard: generally, it's traffic – whether of cars or people – that makes it hard going. This is because everyone is trying to get to work at the same time. So could you shift what time you start and end work? For example, could you start work at seven and end at three rather than the standard nine to five? You would have a more enjoyable commute because you'd be in a smaller group of people traveling to work at those times. Some employers are okay with this kind of arrangement if the team as a whole can cover for one another, so bear in mind that you might need to be flexible too if other members of your team want to do the same: perhaps you can do this two days a week and another three days a week you could come in at the regular time. Perhaps you can also look at working a later shift, such as eleven till seven. Yes, that sounds like a late finish, but you'll have a relaxed start to your day and perhaps on the days when you finish late you can socialise after work – meet friends for a drink, go for dinner, maybe catch a film or a theatre show. It's all about thinking differently.

Better three hours too soon than a
minute too late.

William Shakespeare

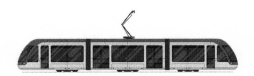

Change how you commute

S O LET'S SAY THAT YOU currently take the metro. Can you bike to work? Walk? Use a commuter ferry if you live and work near a river? Run? That may sound crazy but we had a friend who worked as a project manager at a location that took about an hour to commute to, till he realised that he could actually *run* to work faster than that (it took him about forty minutes, leaving him time to get showered and dressed for work when he got there). As he was a keen marathon runner, this was perfect training for him. His commuting time was the same but he saved money, got his training done, freed up some of his home time for family activities and meanwhile enjoyed the experience. Can you carpool – to save money and have a more enjoyable journey to work? Think about your commute and whether it can be done in an entirely different way.

When we are no longer able to change
a situation - we are challenged to
change ourselves.

Viktor E. Frankl

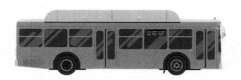

One last thought

I HOPE YOU HAVE ENJOYED READING this book, that some of the suggestions are useful to you and make your commute happier. Your commuting needs will undoubtedly change over time. You'll get a different job, a different home, you'll have friends and family, a partner or kids to include in your traveling plans. Your need for certain things will change over time too: perhaps right now you crave excitement and exercise but will come to value some peace and serenity later on before deciding the time has come for something new along your journey. You may go through this book, make some changes and be happier with your commute – I certainly hope so! But do come back to this book from time to time and see whether your needs and desires have changed and if so, what changes you need to make in response. Look out for new gadgets, new apps, new ideas (I'm pretty sure I haven't thought of everything) to help you out. Revise your commute from time to time or it will get dull again. Remember always that your commute is *yours*.

You can also visit my Pinterest page to view the board for this book if you'd like to see ideas that might make your commute easier, from products to books as well as some funnies: www.pinterest.com/melissaaddey

If you enjoyed this book and have a moment to spare (while commuting, of course!) then I would really appreciate a review on the site where you bought it. Thank you for your help.

Good luck and happy travels!

The only journey is the one within.

Rainer Maria Rilke

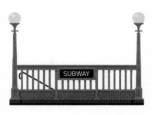

Your Free Book

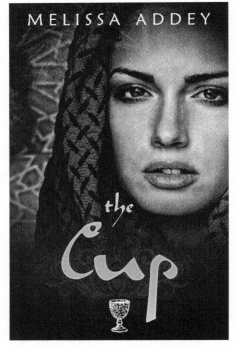

The city of Kairouan in Tunisia, 1020. Hela has powers too strong for a child – both to feel the pain of those around her and to heal them. But when she is given a mysterious cup by a slave woman, its powers overtake her life, forcing her into a vow she cannot hope to keep. So begins a quartet of historical novels set in Morocco as the Almoravid Dynasty sweeps across Northern Africa and Spain, creating a Muslim Empire that endured for generations.

Download your free copy at
www.melissaaddey.com

Commuter studies for further reading

I N CASE YOU WANTED TO read up on what commuting does to you.

Commuters with 45+ min commutes each way reported lower sleep quality and more exhaustion than those with shorter commutes: *The Regus Work-Life Balance Index for 2012. Published on May 08, 2012*

Commuters showed higher blood sugar, blood pressure and cholesterol levels as well as higher tendency toward depression, anxiety, and social isolation: *Commuting Distance, Cardiorespiratory Fitness, and Metabolic Risk. Hoehner, Christine M. et al. American Journal of Preventive Medicine, Volume 42, Issue 6, 571 - 578*

Commuters reported higher levels of stress and anxiety as well as lower life satisfaction and happiness than people with no commutes: *Commuting and Personal Well-being, 2014: Office of National Statistics, UK. Pub 12 Feb 2014*

Commuters 40% more likely to divorce: *Til Work Do Us Part: The Social Fallacy of Long-distance Commuting by Erika Sandow, Urban Studies February 2014 51: 526-543, first published on August 7, 2013*

Social isolation in commuters: *Putnam, Robert D. (2000). Bowling Alone: The Collapse and Revival of American Community. New York: Simon & Schuster*

Obesity, neck and back problems in commuters: *Wellbeing Lower Among Workers With Long Commutes by Steve Crabtree: Gallup-Healthways Well-Being Index 2010*

58% of commuters have experienced road rage, and nearly one in ten commuters have gotten into a fight with another commuter: *Report released by Career Builder based on a survey conducted online within the U.S. by Harris Interactive which polled 3,892 U.S. workers (employed full-time, not self-employed, non-government) ages 18 and over between May 14 and June 4, 2012.*

Reading negative news stories has been proven to make you sadder and more anxious, as well as more likely to exacerbate your own personal worries and anxieties: *Johnston, W. M. and Davey, G. C. L. (1997), The psychological impact of negative TV news bulletins: The catastrophizing of personal worries. British Journal of Psychology, 88: 85–91.*

Biography

I mainly write historical fiction, and am currently writing two series set in very different eras: China in the 1700s and Morocco/Spain in the 1000s. You can download a novella for free on my website: www.MelissaAddey.com

I worked in business for fifteen years before becoming a fulltime writer, during which time I developed new products and packaging for a major supermarket and mentored over 500 entrepreneurs for a government grant-making innovation programme. In 2016 I was made the Leverhulme Trust Writer in Residence at the British Library, which included writing two books, *Merchandise for Authors* and *The Storytelling Entrepreneur*. You can read more about my non-fiction books on my website.

I am currently studying for a PhD in Creative Writing at the University of Surrey.

I love using my writing to interact with people and run regular workshops at the British Library as well as coaching other writers on a one-to-one basis.

I live in London with my husband and two children.

For more information, visit my website
www.melissaaddey.com

Current and forthcoming books include:

Historical Fiction
China
The Consorts
The Fragrant Concubine
The Garden of Perfect Brightness
The Cold Palace

Morocco
The Cup
A String of Silver Beads
None Such as She
Do Not Awaken Love

Picture Books for Children
Kameko and the Monkey-King

Non-Fiction
The Storytelling Entrepreneur
Merchandise for Authors
The Happy Commuter
100 Things to Do while Breastfeeding

Thank you!

A BIG THANK YOU TO THE commuters who made this book better with their interesting commutes, ideas, feedback and a helping hand when needed. Angela, Camilla, Carlo, Christina, Etain, Ina, Little Emma, Helen, Jason, Roberto and Ryan. And to Streetlight Graphics, for making imaginary things real and beautiful, as ever.

79883753R00149